The

Weight Maintenance

Survival Guide

Kelly D. Brownell, Ph.D.
University of Pennsylvania School of Medicine

Judith Rodin, Ph.D.
Yale University

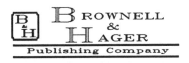

BROWNELL
&
HAGER
Publishing Company

Dallas   Philadelphia

Library of Congress Catalog Card Number:

90-93239

ISBN 1-878513-01-X

Address orders to:

        The LEARN™ Education Center
        1555 W. Mockingbird Lane, Suite 203
        Dallas, Texas 75235

        In Dallas (214) 637-7700
        Or Toll-Free 1-800-736-READ
        Fax Number (214) 637-0529

Permission to reprint cartoons was granted by the Universal Press Syndicate, Chronicle Features, *The Washington Post*, and the United Features Syndicate, Inc.

TABLE OF CONTENTS

CHAPTER ONE

Introduction: Kicking Off A New Life

Welcome to a new life! This program is for a lifetime. You've made a real commitment to getting in control of your weight. This is the program that will help you maintain your weight.

Through our clinical work, and our travels around the world speaking about problems of weight, we hear a single common cry. The major problem faced by people who succeed in losing weight is that they cannot maintain the losses.

Doctors used to doubt their patients when they heard how difficult it was to keep weight off. Now we know that people go up and down repeatedly, through many cycles of gaining and losing, because they simply don't know how to maintain a constant weight. Most people have spent their lives either being on a diet or letting it all go. They have no experience with that "middle ground."

What is Maintenance?

Let's begin by defining maintenance. Maintenance is keeping your weight at some steady or stable point. For some people that means setting an absolute number and sticking to it. But for most people, maintenance is keeping weight within a range, for example, 165 to 168 pounds or 125 to 135 pounds. For other people maintenance is keeping within a particular size or set of clothes.

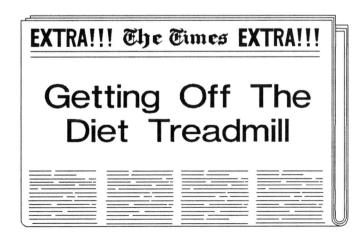

EXTRA!!! The Times EXTRA!!!

Getting Off The Diet Treadmill

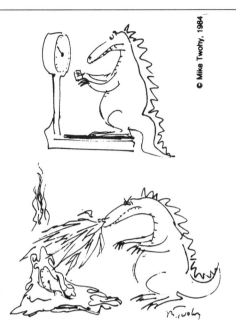

© Mike Twohy, 1984

Is This Book For You?

This guide is for everyone who wants to give up a lifetime of dieting and regaining. It is for everyone whose goal is to keep weight balanced and to prevent dieting from ruling their life. You may already be at a weight that you are comfortable with. You've lost weight and you don't want to be on a diet for the rest of your life. You are ready for maintenance now. Or, perhaps maintenance is still a more distant goal and you have more weight to lose. This book will help you lose that weight -- **permanently.** You should not use this book, however, if you are only dieting for a particular day or event. Many people lose weight for their daughter's wedding, or for their class reunion, and don't really have long-term maintenance as a goal. If that's you, you will probably not find this book to be very helpful.

Maintenance History Questionnaire

Many people lose weight many times only to regain. Often they put on a few extra pounds with each new cycle. Does this sound all too familiar? The questionnaire beginning on the opposite page is useful in pointing out the problems you have had with weight maintenance in the past. Take a few minutes now to complete the eight questions.

Now that you have completed the questionnaire, let's look at your answer to question 1. If you haven't been able to keep yourself at a steady or stable weight for longer than one year, you probably have never gotten your body to adjust, biochemically and psychologically, to a particular weight. Weight maintenance gets easier after a year or so because of the way your body adapts. This program is designed to stabilize your weight over the long haul.

Maintenance History Questionnaire

1. What is the longest period of time you have ever kept yourself at a steady or stable weight? _____ months.

2. How many times in your life would you estimate you have LOST the number of pounds shown below? For example, if you have lost 30 pounds twice, you would put a check in the column marked 1-2 times. Please answer for each weight category.

	0 times	1-2	3-5	6-10	11-15	16-20	21-25	26+
1 - 5 lbs	____	____	____	____	____	____	____	____
6 -10 lbs	____	____	____	____	____	____	____	____
11-20 lbs	____	____	____	____	____	____	____	____
21-30 lbs	____	____	____	____	____	____	____	____
31-50 lbs	____	____	____	____	____	____	____	____
51 + lbs	____	____	____	____	____	____	____	____

3. How many times in your life would you estimate you have GAINED BACK the number of pounds shown below? For example, if you have gained back 30 pounds twice, you would put a check in the column marked 1-2 times. Please answer for each weight category.

	0 times	1-2	3-5	6-10	11-15	16-20	21-25	26+
1 - 5 lbs	____	____	____	____	____	____	____	____
6 -10 lbs	____	____	____	____	____	____	____	____
11-20 lbs	____	____	____	____	____	____	____	____
21-30 lbs	____	____	____	____	____	____	____	____
31-50 lbs	____	____	____	____	____	____	____	____
51 + lbs	____	____	____	____	____	____	____	____

4. How much of the time are you dieting?

____Never   ____Rarely   ____Sometimes   ____Frequently   ____Almost always

Maintenance History Questionnaire (continued)

5.   How often do you feel like you give too much conscious thought and attention to food?

___Never   ___Rarely   ___Sometimes   ___Frequently   ___Almost always

6.   How often do you feel guilty when you eat your favorite high calorie foods?

___Never   ___Rarely   ___Sometimes   ___Frequently   ___Almost always

7.   How often do you wish you could eat "like normal people do"?

___Never   ___Rarely   ___Sometimes   ___Frequently   ___Almost always

8.   How often do you hate yourself when you gain weight?

___Never   ___Rarely   ___Sometimes   ___Frequently   ___Almost always

Now look at your answer to questions 2 and 3. The more cycles of dieting and regaining you have been through, the more difficult dieting has probably become for you. If you feel like it's gotten easier to regain and harder to lose, you're right. The number of cycles you've been through may be the culprit. This program will help you get off the weight cycling seesaw. If you stay on the seesaw, you may find it more difficult to control your weight later.

The next five questions all deal with your food and weight preoccupations. The more of these questions you answer "frequently" or "almost always," the more this program will help. Diet and weight preoccupation are not the answer. In fact, they are counterproductive. There are very different approaches needed to maintain weight than to lose weight. Your frequent worries and concerns, as indicated by these five questions, suggest that you can benefit greatly from learning the right maintenance strategies.

Won't it be great to have days, weeks, months even, when you won't have to worry about your weight and be preoccupied with your eating?! That's what this program is all about.

Why Is This Program Different?

How will this be different from other books and programs? Surprisingly, there are very few maintenance programs and almost no books on the subject. Everybody seems focused on weight loss; perhaps because so many of us have to do it so many times. So there aren't many places you can turn to learn about the right maintenance techniques and strategies. That's why we believe this book is so important and why we decided to write it.

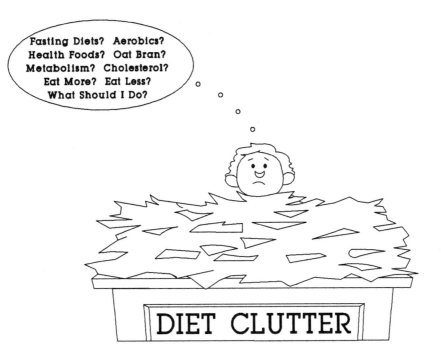

As you go through the program, some of the techniques will be familiar to you, but they are used in a different way when focusing on maintenance rather than weight loss. Others will be totally new techniques or new ways of thinking about yourself, your body, your weight or food. Some of these ideas may seem foreign. "What does it mean to learn how to eat my favorite high calorie foods? I know too well how to eat them. That's what gets me into trouble," you complain. But we'll teach you how because now you are focusing on **the rest of your life**.

You may feel swamped by all the weight control information you've read in your lifetime. This book is simply written, definitive and easy to work through. If you follow the principles covered here you can:

- **Break the diet mentality**
- **Learn to establish a reasonable weight goal**
- **Prevent relapse**
- **Change unhelpful thoughts and feelings**
- **Develop a more flexible lifestyle**
- **Enjoy your new changes**
- **Decrease the time and effort you spend worrying about food and weight**

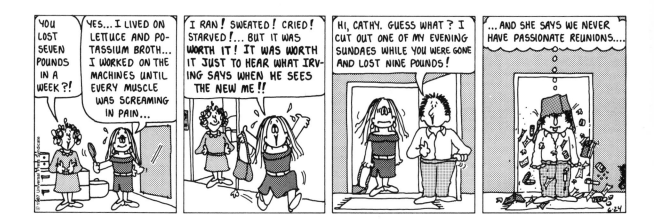

How Do You Feel About Yourself?

On the following page we have provided a simple "What I Like About Me" quiz for you to complete. Please take a few minutes now the complete the scale.

Feeling good about yourself and what you do is an important springboard for maintenance. We will explore this further with you in the chapters that follow, and will show that there is more to life than weight. Helping you put your weight in the proper perspective is one of the fundamental steps to successful weight maintenance.

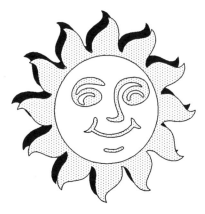

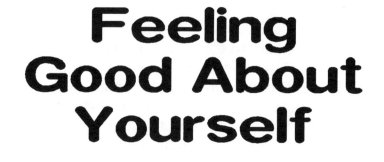

"What I Like About Me" Scale

Please consider how important each of the dimensions listed here is to your sense of self-worth. Give each item a rating between 1 and 100: If an item is of utmost importance to how you feel about yourself, give it a 100; if an item is of absolutely no importance to how you feel about yourself, give it a 1. Use the numbers in-between to reflect varying degrees of importance. You can use the numbers as often as you like (e.g., you can give more than one item a rating of 100).

_____ feeling intelligent   _____ having good friends

_____ excelling at work or school   _____ being physically coordinated

_____ being a good child   _____ being altruistic

_____ feeling attractive   _____ being creative

_____ caring about social causes   _____ having a romantic partner

_____ doing well at athletic activities _____ being a good parent

_____ being politically active

Others: (specify)

_____ _____   _____ _____

_____ _____   _____ _____

Who Are The Authors?

We are both professors and researchers and run programs for people with eating and weight problems. Kelly Brownell is a Professor in the Department of Psychiatry at the University of Pennsylvania School of Medicine, and Judith Rodin is a Professor of Psychology, Psychiatry and Medicine at Yale University. We have done research for almost twenty years in the area of weight control and weight maintenance. We have both written books on the topic and published several hundred articles in scientific journals. It is this combination of our clinical and research experience that makes us see how greatly this book is needed. People we encounter in our programs, in our lectures, or in our appearance on television and radio shows tell us how there is abundant help for the person who wants to lose weight, but almost nothing on maintaining weight. This prompted us to team together to prepare this book.

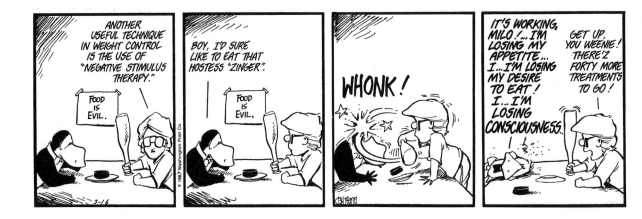

CHAPTER TWO

Cultural Ideals, Body Ideals

The "Right" Look

Billions of dollars are spent each year beautifying our bodies. Estimates show that Americans spend more on looking good than on education or social services. An overwhelming number of women in particular believe they are to heavy.

Did you ever stop to think about where these feelings come from? Do other people's values have you in their grip?

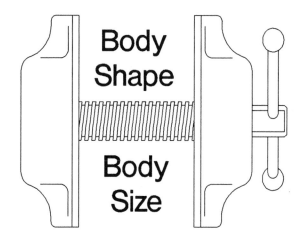

Modern technology has made a dramatic impact on our body image. Mass retailing and machine-produced clothing -- promoted by extensive advertising -- have given us a single "look." Televisions in every house make beautiful people seem like friends and neighbors.

Cultural Beauty Ideals

Why do people feel the way they do about weight? We believe that cultural ideals about beauty are the culprit. You may not be able to set a realistic weight goal unless you stand face-to-face with this reality.

Appearance matters in our society -- to an extraordinary extent. We are worried about how we look because physical appearance seems so important to happiness. Attractiveness equals success, power, and acceptance. Americans believe that what is beautiful is good. These attitudes develop early. Preschool children view attractive friends as friendlier and smarter than unattractive children. Physical attractiveness is related to popularity, even in the preschool classroom.

Thinness Equals Beauty. Thin is in! In fact, the trend has been for the ideal of beauty to get thinner and thinner. Looking at the measurements of contestants in the Miss America pageant since 1959, there has been a striking decrease in body weight and size. Since 1970, the winners have usually been the thinnest of the five finalists. Similarly, the body sizes of Playboy Magazine centerfold models have greatly decreased over recent years. We don't want to be thin and soft, however. The look for the 90's is fit and muscular.

People are more preoccupied and less satisfied with their bodies now than ever. They judge themselves and others more harshly for not measuring up to some ideal standard.

Cultural Beauty Ideals

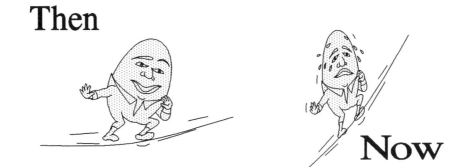

Then

Now

How We Feel About Our Bodies

In 1987, *Psychology Today* Magazine surveyed its readers' feelings about appearance and weight. A full 88% were concerned enough with their appearance to do something about it. Of course people who choose to return a survey on body image may be likely to care more than most about their appearance. But the results of this survey are similar to those that have recently been found in studies where the participants are selected at random. People feel intense pressure to look good.

An earlier survey on body image was published in *Psychology Today* in 1972. People in the 1970's were considerably more satisfied with their bodies than people are today. Men especially seem more concerned about how they look now than they used to. But for both sexes, the pressure to look good has intensified in the last 15 years.

Consider the table below comparing the two surveys. Our dissatisfaction has grown for every area of our bodies.

UNHAPPY BODIES

People Dissatisfied with Body Areas or Dimensions

	1972 Survey				1987 Survey	
	Men	Women			Men	Women
Height	13%	13%		Height	20%	17%
Weight	35	48		Weight	41	55
Muscle Tone	25	30		Muscle Tone	32	55
Overall Face	8	11		Face	20	20
Breast/Chest	18	26		Upper Torso	28	32
Abdomen	36	50		Mid Torso	50	7
Hips/Upper Thighs	12	49		Lower Torso	21	50
Overall				"Looks As		
Appearance	15	25		They Are"	34	38

The survey also shows how important weight is to body image. Over 40% of the men and 50% of the women were unhappy with their weight in 1987. Men were most dissatisfied with their bellies and women with their thighs. These are the areas most often affected by weight gain for each sex.

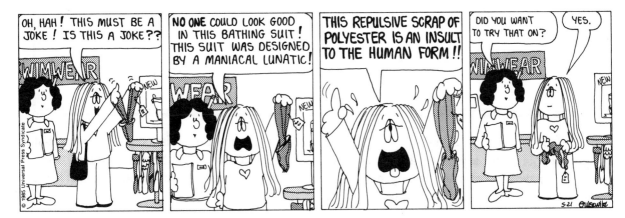

Rating Your Body Satisfaction

Do you feel caught by your own body dissatisfaction? Answer the following questions to learn more about how you view your body.

Rate how you feel about each aspect of your body according to the following code:

7 = strong positive feeling
6 = positive feeling
5 = slight positive feeling
4 = have no feeling one way or the other
3 = slight negative feeling
2 = negative feeling
1 = strong negative feeling

How Do You Feel About Your Body?

My Looks - Just The Way They Are   _____

Height   _____

Weight   _____

Chest or Breasts   _____

Waist   _____

Stomach   _____

Hips   _____

Thighs   _____

Buttocks   _____

Calves   _____

TOTAL SCORE   _____

On this scale, the lower your score on each item, the more dissatisfied you are with that part of your body. If your total score (the answers to all ten added together) is between 10 and 20, you have a very negative body image. Many of the exercises and techniques you will learn in this book deal with ways to improve your body image.

What is Body Image?

Many people are dissatisfied with how they look because their ideal is so far from how they think they look at the present time. A good way to determine your own judgments are to use the set of figures on the following page. These figures are adapted from ones developed by University of Pennsylvania psychiatrist Albert J. Stunkard and psychologist Paul Rozin and their colleagues. They are now widely used as research tools to investigate body image, and body image differences between men and women.

Body Image Exercise

Find the set of figures for your sex. Working first with the array of drawings of figures from the **head to waist,** choose the number below the figure which best illustrates:

a) How you think you currently look. Choose the figure that best represents your actual size.
    Figure #_____

b) Choose the figure that best represents how you would like to look (your ideal figure).
    Figure #_____

c) Choose the figure that best represents how you think others see you.
    Figure #_____

d) Choose the figure that you think best represents what is most attractive to the opposite sex.
    Figure #_____

Now, repeat the same procedure for the figures from waist to feet.

a) How you think you currently look. Choose the figure that best represents your actual size.
    Figure #_____

b) Choose the figure that best represents how you would like to look (your ideal figure).
    Figure #_____

c) Choose the figure that best represents how you think others see you.
    Figure #_____

d) Choose the figure that you think best represents what is most attractive to the opposite sex.
    Figure#_____

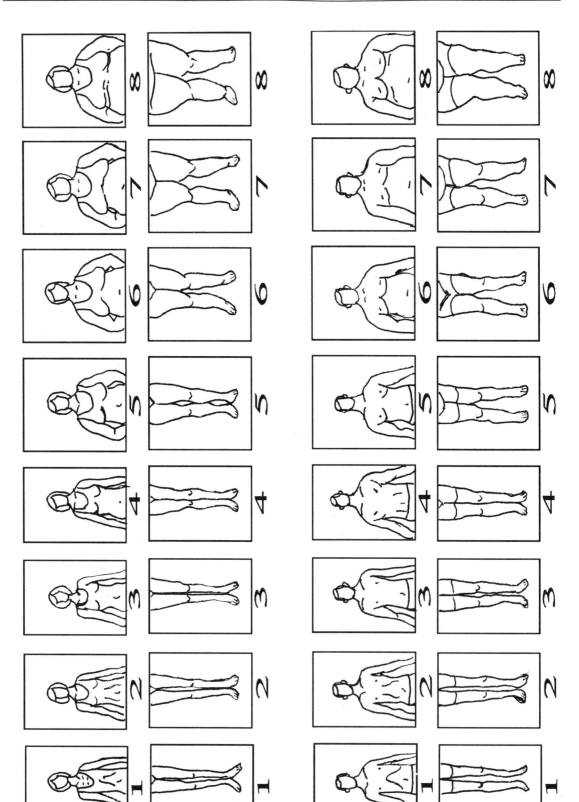

Since each figure has a number associated with it, you can calculate your body image scores. For example, the numerical difference between your view of how you think you look and how you would like to look (the answer to "a" compared to the answer to "b") represents your self/ideal discrepancy. Or, the difference between your ideal and your view of what the opposite sex finds attractive represents the extent to which your ideal is even more extreme (and perhaps harder to attain) than what the opposite sex expects of you.

In studies we and others have done, the majority of people -- both males and females -- have an ideal figure in mind that's different from how they think they actually look. What's different between men and women is simply the direction of the discrepancy. Men are as likely to express a desire to be heavier as to be thinner. In contrast, very few women want to be heavier. Almost all women choose an ideal figure that is thinner than their perceived figure. In other words, men and women seem equally unhappy with their bodies, but unlike men, women are unanimous in their desire to be thinner.

Body Esteem/Self Esteem

Why is it so important to understand how you view your body, and to change it? People who see a great difference between how their bodies look and how they think they **ought** to look, have lower self esteem. They feel worse about themselves in general, not only about their body and weight. They also tend to have more eating problems. Changing the way that you think about your body is going to be central to your weight maintenance efforts.

Remember that people are affected by their body image because of the emphasis society places on our bodies. We are forced to ask ourselves, "Am I attractive enough?" When women enter a room they often look around to see who is thinner, so they can decide where they stand. People in our society ask "Is my body impressing others and winning their approval?" We feel on-stage, observed and scrutinized. This increases the importance of visible parts of the body that are subject to immediate public scrutiny. Weight, of course, is the most central of these. On the other hand, the notion that the body is infinitely changeable is problematic when it comes to weight.

Body Size: Whose Choice Is It?

Our genes contribute a lot to determining our body size and weight. Research on heredity and weight has shown that identical twins have body weights over twice as similar as non-identical twins or siblings. When identical twins are raised apart, they still have weights that are far more similar than either non-identical twins or siblings reared together.

Genes limit our ability to shape the bodies we would like. However, despite the limitations of our genetic determination, we are made to feel ashamed and guilty if we fall short of cultural weight ideals.

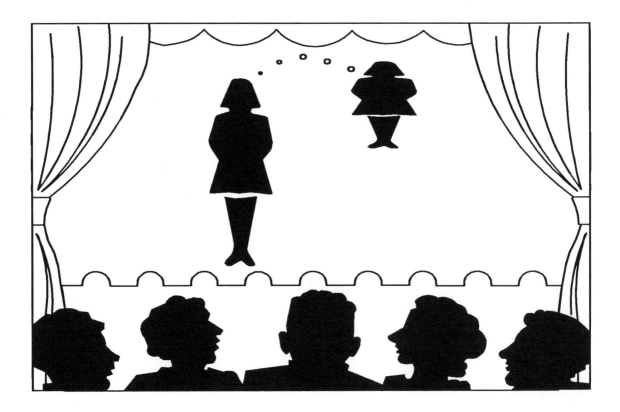

Women Are Fatter Than Men. Women start out in life with more fat then men do. This difference increases over the life cycle.

Imposed by nature, women's bodies are equipped to promote the development of fat cells and the storage of body fat. Fat is important for the ability to bear children. Regardless of what country or time period they have lived in, women have had more fat than men, on the average. Remember that fat and weight are different. Fat refers to the amount of body fat you have; the body also has muscle and water. People of the same weight can differ dramatically in body fat.

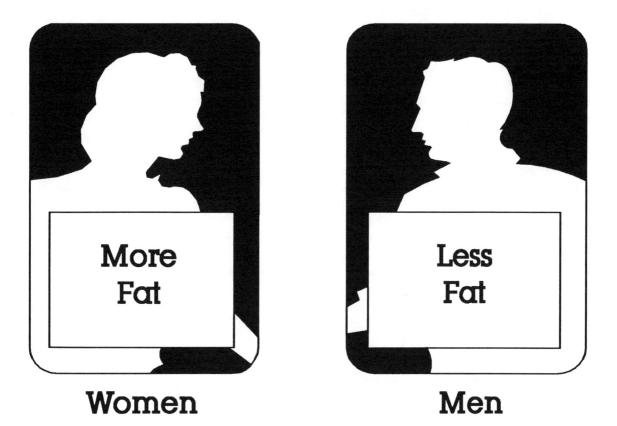

Setting Realistic Weight Goals

What is a realistic weight goal? You may be poised for trouble if your ideal weight is something your genes and biology will never let you achieve. The ideal pushed by society (through models, actors, ads, etc.) may be impossible for you or almost anyone to achieve.

Models and actors have beauty as their career. They spend an enormous amount of time working out and taking care of their physical appearance. When the 1989 Miss America contestants were interviewed, all of them said they exercised, some as many as 34 hours a week. All of them admitted to **constantly** watching what they eat. For the average person, this is not only impossible, given the rest of the demands on their lives, but may be psychologically unhealthy.

To maintain your weight you need to set a realistic weight goal. Don't picture Miss America, the model on television, or even the friend down the street. What weight would be reasonable for **you**? What dress or suit size would make you feel like a normal person? Unless you are gearing up to compete in the Olympics or the Miss America contest, you probably don't need to achieve the ideal held out by society.

Solving The Puzzle

How can you decide on a more **realistic** weight goal? First, make a list of the times when you have felt really happy with yourself, your accomplishments, your life in general. Now write down what you weighed at that time. Do this for as many times in your adult life as you can remember.

Second, what is the largest size of clothes that you feel comfortable in? What size are you wearing when you can look in the mirror and say "I look pretty good." Think about the times when you could say "This looks really great considering where I've been." What weight do you have to be to wear that size?

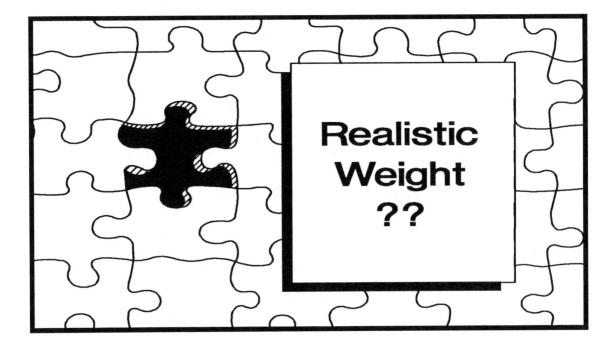

Third, think about a friend or family member who looks "normal" to you. Not the models and the movie stars, but someone you know. Pick somebody who is around the same age and has the same body frame as yours. Ask them what they weigh and use it as data in setting your own realistic goal.

When you finish these exercises, you should have a weight, or better yet a weight range, in mind. This should be considered your realistic weight goal.

Am I Really OK? Suppose you can reach and maintain the realistic weight goal you just set for yourself. It may be heavier than your ideal, but your ideal is probably out of line. Try this exercise to see if being thinner than this realistic weight would really matter.

Go back to the chart you filled out in Chapter 1 called the "What I Like About Me Scale." Imagine yourself **10 pounds lighter than the realistic weight goal** you just picked. Would any of your ratings change?

If no, you have found a realistic, comfortable target weight.

If yes, you have diagnosed the areas where your self-esteem is linked too closely to your body weight. Remember, society makes you feel this way. Now is the time for change.

Your realistic weight goal is the weight at which you could feel good about how you look. This may be higher than you had been hoping. When you have an unrealistic ideal, you feel ashamed. Interestingly, the word shame derives from the word, to cover, so shame is strongly related to the desire to hide and cover up. It is time to take the cover off and help you get rid of the shame. This is how maintenance works.

Now Is The Time
For Change

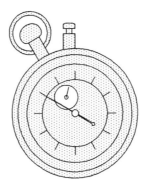

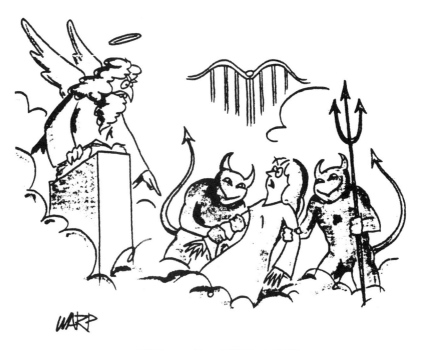

"It's because I have fat thighs, isn't it!"

CHAPTER THREE

Risk Assessment

How Much Control Do You Have?

How would you characterize your hold on eating and your weight? Fill out the Control Quiz on the following page and we will show you how to use your responses to spot danger before it arrives.

Control is a major issue for people with weight and eating problems. Some people feel they have great control but actually don't, while others fear they have no control but do well. There are two issues here -- how much control you have and how much control you **think** you have.

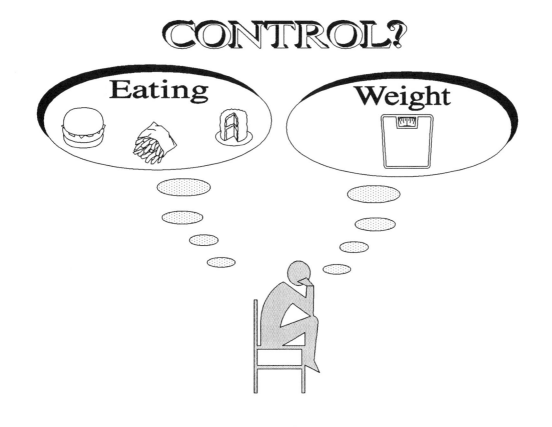

Control Quiz

1. **How fearful are you that you will regain weight?**

    Not At All   Slightly   Somewhat   Quite   Extremely

2. **Do certain foods make you lose control?**

    Not At All   A Little   To Some Extent   Usually   Absolutely

3. **How vulnerable do you feel to the possibility of losing control over your eating?**

    Not At All   Slightly   Somewhat   Quite   Extremely

4. **When you are faced by situations where you are likely to overeat, how often can you control yourself?**

    Always   Usually   Sometimes   Rarely   Never

5. **For what percentage of the times you eat would you say you eat reasonably and under control?**

    100%   75%   50%   25%   0%

6. **Overall, how much control would you say you have over eating?**

    Complete   Moderate   Some   A Little   None

It is important for you to consider control over both **eating** and **weight**. Some people control their weight even though their control over eating is tenuous. They might eat out of control at times and then "make up for it" by severely restricting their eating at other times. Weight may stay stable, but eating is erratic. Other people are able to restrict their eating much of the time, but are extremely fearful of gaining weight. When looking over your responses to the Control Quiz, try to separate in your mind how much control you actually have, how much control you feel you have, and how the issue of control might be different for eating and weight.

The first three questions on the Control Quiz address your **perception** of control. Your responses to these will show how much control you **feel** you have and how vulnerable you may be. High scores on these questions indicate that you are fearful of losing control. This fear may make you feel vulnerable, which in turn can sap a lot of your mental energy. Note that question 1 deals with your fear of gaining weight, while questions 2 and 3 deal with control over eating. Being specific about perceived and actual control is important for later parts of the program.

The last three questions on the Control Quiz deal with how much control you **actually** have. High scores on these show that you have trouble controlling your eating, probably in response to a number of factors. Examples of these factors would be physical conditions such as fatigue, moods such as anger or loneliness, or environmental situations such as being exposed to food.

Overestimating your control can be a problem because you can be complacent and may expose yourself to temptation when avoidance would be a better tactic. People who feel this way are not as vigilant as they need be.

The opposite side of the coin is the person who actually has control but feels vulnerable. As an example, the two of us, along with Dr. Jack Wilmore from the University of Texas, did a survey in **Runner's World** magazine. After tabulating several thousand responses, we found that 48% of women and 21% of men reported being "terrified" about being overweight. Considering that readers of **Runner's World** are likely to be more fit than the population in general, these are striking numbers. Certainly not this many people actually have such fragile control to justify the terror they feel, so this serves as an example of people who may have better control than they believe.

It is important that your actual control and perceived control come into line. This can be done by making an honest assessment of your feelings of vulnerability and your actual control. Being terrorized is not desirable, but nor is being complacent. Feelings of vulnerability are natural, but are still unpleasant. The good news is that it can change. In fact, one of the primary aims for this book is to give you the confidence that you can handle anything.

Poised on the Edge

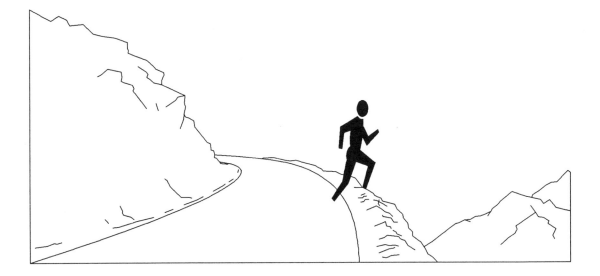

Poised on The Edge of a Cliff

We will use the example of a cliff to make a point. Many dieters, even those who have lost weight and kept if off for years, feel like they are poised on the edge of a cliff. Their balance is so precarious that the least little error sends them tumbling over the edge. Once the fall begins, there is no return.

One wonders how weeks or even months of successful dieting can be undone by a minor push, but the sad truth for many dieters is that a small nudge can do it. Eating one forbidden food, gaining weight when you expect to lose, or letting loose and feeling out of control can send a person off the cliff.

Here is a place where maintainers differ from one another. One person might have a very tenuous hold on eating, so that minor events signal the end. Another person might have much more control and almost nothing will derail their progress. This book is designed to make you feel like the second person.

Navigating Your Way To Freedom

You **can** steer a course that will give you freedom from feeling vulnerable, and freedom from the fear that loss of control is only a step away. Think of the relief this can be.

There are two ways to avoid the problems with cliffs. One is to stay away from cliffs. As silly as this sounds, this philosophy is central to successful maintenance. By navigating a safe course, you can avoid situations in which you are vulnerable. The key to this is risk assessment.

The second important step is to fortify yourself with skills, so that you can withstand pressures to topple over the cliffs you can't avoid. Having these skills will increase your confidence that **you** are in control, which will go a long way to making you the master of your weight.

Let's take an example to show these two key steps. Marie is doing well on her diet but is invited to a baby shower. The shower will be hosted by a woman who loves to bake delicious desserts. Marie knows in advance that the shower is a high-risk situation, so we could call it a cliff. If she eats the delicious desserts, she might fall from the cliff and leave her diet behind. Using the two approaches discussed above, here is how Marie could deal with this risky setting.

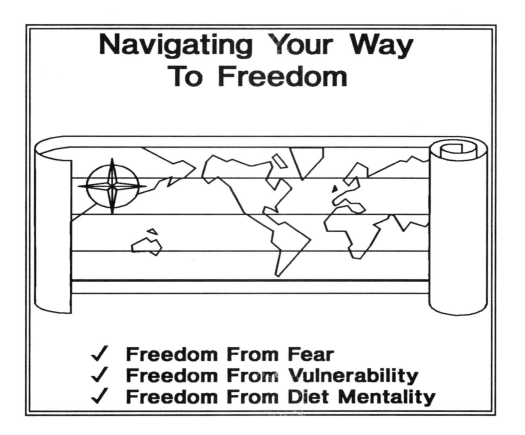

Strategy #1

Marie could avoid the shower. If she feels vulnerable and believes that she would almost certainly lose control, then she must make the decision of whether the shower or her weight is more important. The problem with this approach is that Marie may feel resentful when she has to avoid important and enjoyable activities. Therefore, we do not recommend that she employ this strategy too often. However, some situations can and should be avoided because the risk is too high.

Strategy #2

Strategy #2 involves preplanning and problem-solving. Marie can take certain actions to see that the shower does not become her diet cliff. As one example, she could have a big salad just before she goes, and could fill up on non-caloric beverages once she arrives. She could tell a friend that she is trying to watch the calories so that they might share a single dessert. She could make sure that she sits in a section of the room where the desserts are least accessible. In doing these things, Marie would not lose control.

There are many more examples of what Marie might do to avoid overeating in this situation. These will be discussed later, but we give you this example to show that Marie could increase her chances of successful weight maintenance by charting a course **before** the situation occurs. She would feel better and in control. When setting out on a journey that will bring you face-to-face with danger, it is best to be prepared, to have a plan, and to chart a defined course.

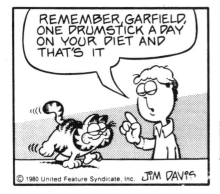 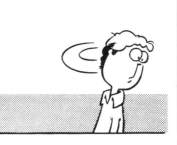 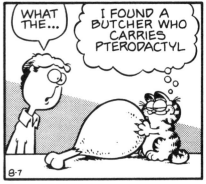

What Is Risk?

Risk occurs when you are in a situation where you are likely to make mistakes, to err, to go off your program. Your feelings of vulnerability are increased. Temptation is present, and you realize from your past experiences that the situation is fragile.

What is risky for one dieter is risk-free for another. Being at a cocktail party with cheese and crackers may be murder for someone who craves cheese, but for a cheese hater, control is no problem. Alcohol can weaken control for one person but not another. For some, specific foods can create risk (think of a food where you can never eat just one bite), but for others it may be a mood (being lonely, depressed), a physical state (fatigue), or a social situation (everyone else is eating).

What Is Risk Assessment?

Risk assessment is self-awareness. It is knowing the exact conditions that make you vulnerable. "But wait!" you say. "I already know this from years of dieting experience." It is true that you know more than anyone, but there is still much to learn. By the time we finish, you will be an expert on understanding risk, and how to spot risk. But most important, you will now learn what your years of dieting experience haven't taught you -- how to minimize the danger from risky situations.

Because risk is highly individual, the key is to learn how to identify risk and then to apply this knowledge to your own situation. The guidelines which follow will help you do just this.

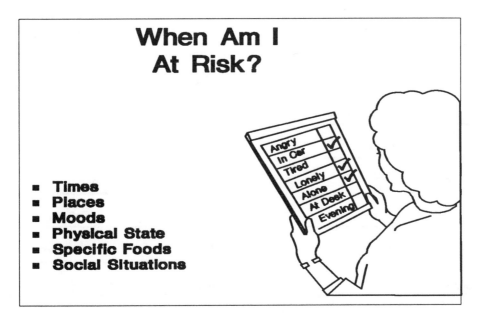

Charting Your High-Risk Situations

Take a few minutes now to complete the chart on the opposite page entitled "My Own Risk Factors." But first, look over the sample chart we have provided below. This shows some of the common themes that emerge in the people we work with. Your chart need not look like this, but the sample chart will give you some idea of how a person might respond.

As you complete the blank chart, think carefully about the situations that give you trouble. Think back over past diets and past maintenance experiences to identify the factors that make you eat more than you want.

As you are thinking about what to put in the chart, consider the factors that influence your control. These could be certain moods, certain foods, social situations, places, or any other factors you feel are relevant.

Next to where you list the situation, think about the aspects of the situation that create risk. Is it the taste of a food? Maybe eating generates good feelings like relaxation. Maybe the situation creates risk because good food is too available.

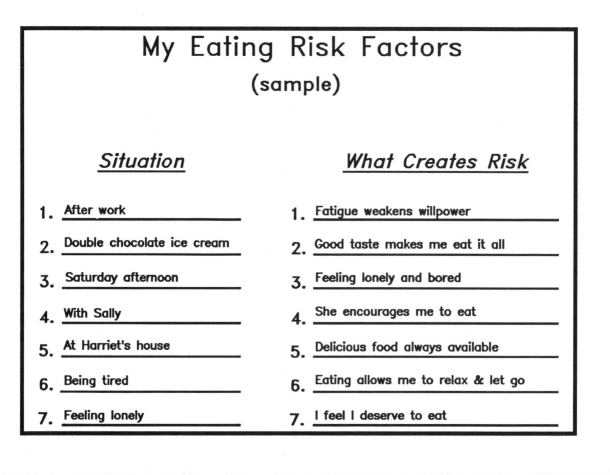

My Eating Risk Factors
(sample)

Situation	_What Creates Risk_
1. After work	1. Fatigue weakens willpower
2. Double chocolate ice cream	2. Good taste makes me eat it all
3. Saturday afternoon	3. Feeling lonely and bored
4. With Sally	4. She encourages me to eat
5. At Harriet's house	5. Delicious food always available
6. Being tired	6. Eating allows me to relax & let go
7. Feeling lonely	7. I feel I deserve to eat

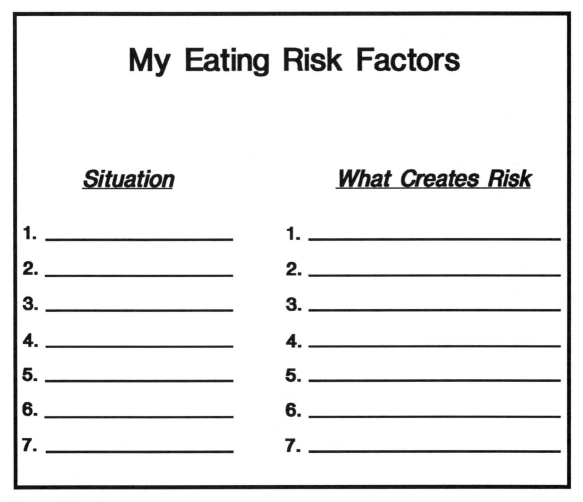

My Eating Risk Factors

Situation	*What Creates Risk*
1. _____	1. _____
2. _____	2. _____
3. _____	3. _____
4. _____	4. _____
5. _____	5. _____
6. _____	6. _____
7. _____	7. _____

Record Keeping

For the next three weeks, fill out the Risk Record every day. Make photocopies of the Risk Record or draw your own by hand, and then complete one for each day. The Risk Record will form a chronicle of your eating, will help you identify the situations in which risk is high, and will help you learn what it is about some situations that makes them risky.

The Risk Record contains space for listing the food you eat, the time, place, mood, physical state, social situation, and comments about what created the risk. Fill in each of the columns and pay attention to whether patterns emerge.

You do not need to write down every food you eat in the Risk Record. The purpose of the record is to help you analyze situations that create risk. This may or may not involve excess eating. For example, eating an apple and yogurt for breakfast need not be entered, if breakfast is not a high-risk situation for you. Going out to lunch with coworkers may be a high-risk situation even if you don't overdo it on a certain day. If the situation has been risky in the past, if you are eating a problem food, if the people you are around encourage you to eat, or if the way you feel creates risk, put it in the record.

After keeping the Risk Record for three weeks, go back and amend your chart of risk factors. What did you learn from three weeks of keeping the records that will help you make a better list? You might want to do this every six months or so to make sure new risk situations haven't crept into your life. We talk in Chapters 10 and 12 about reevaluating your risk situations, and in Chapter 5 we discuss the need for periodic "check-ups." Risk assessment is one area where check-ups might be useful.

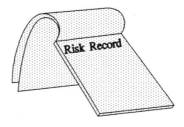

Keep
Risk Record

The Bottom Line

You should be approaching the point where you know exactly what creates risk. You should be able to predict how difficult control will be in any situation. Furthermore, you should know what it is about these situations that creates the risk. This information will be invaluable as we develop special skills so that: 1) You are never surprised by risk; and 2) You are confident you can handle most situations.

In the sections that follow, we will discuss many ways to make use of the information from these risk charts. Changing behavior begins with understanding behavior. In this case, decreasing feelings of vulnerability and increasing confidence begins with understanding risk. Now that you understand, let's move ahead!

Risk Record

Food and Amount Eaten	Time	Place	Mood	Physical State	Social Situation	What Created Risk

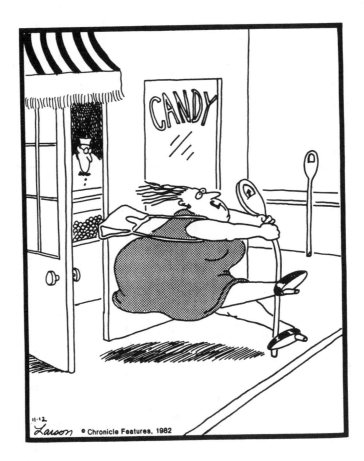

CHAPTER FOUR

Relapse Prevention

What Is Relapse Prevention?

Keeping weight off. These three words sound so simple, yet represent a daunting task to most people. Some individuals, even after months of successful weight maintenance, are terrified they will regain weight. As funny as it sounds, this feeling of vulnerability makes a person more vulnerable. It is like the famous quote from Franklin Roosevelt, "We have nothing to fear but fear itself."

Feelings of vulnerability will go away only after you develop the skills and confidence to handle any situation. Part of this will occur when you understand how to prevent relapse.

Most individuals lose and regain weight a number of times before they finally get the problem solved. Almost everyone has experience with making mistakes, slipping, going back to the old ways, and regaining weight. This is what most people consider "relapse". We can help you prevent it.

The word relapse is well-known to people trying to maintain their weight. In general usage, it means return to the old ways, failure, and giving up. We will use the term differently, as we will discuss shortly. From the very beginning, however, we want to emphasize one point.

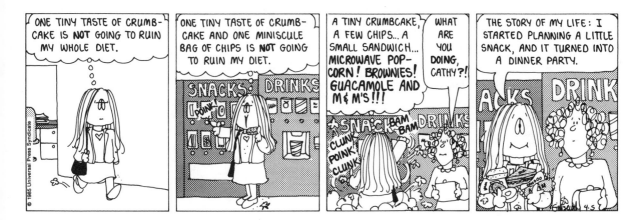

There are many ways to prevent slips and errors, but even the most diligent person will make mistakes. It is the **reaction** to the mistakes that can make or break your program, so we will be working hard on developing a **constructive** response to the inevitable detours you may take as you travel toward permanent weight maintenance.

Part of the challenge is for you to change your mindset. If you break down and have a chocolate croissant when you feel you shouldn't, defining this in your mind as a terrible blunder, a horrible mistake, or an out-of-control error will overstate its importance. This in turn brings guilt and shame, which sets you up for later problems. This chapter will show you how to put these events in perspective and to keep the inevitable detours from sending you reeling off course permanently.

Some Important Words

We believe it is important to use the right terms to describe these matters. We begin with **lapse**. This refers to a slip or mistake, an error or problem with your program. A lapse might be failing to exercise, exceeding your calorie level, eating some food to excess, or slipping from the path you have set for yourself. A lapse is a discreet event. Lapses, of course, can be major or minor, but the first sign of slippage is what we refer to here.

Relapse is when several lapses occur in sequence. If you overeat at one sitting, a lapse has occurred. If you do it a second and third time, you have "re-lapsed". Relapse signals danger, but does not mean losing control completely. It does **not** signal a point of no return. Rather, it simply indicates that the lapses are occurring without interruption. As you can guess, relapse is a signal for vigorous action.

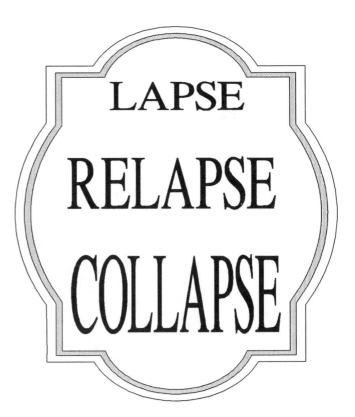

Collapse has obvious meaning. This is when relapse is out of control and there is no hope for return. In the minds of most people, this is when they give up completely and decide they cannot exert control.

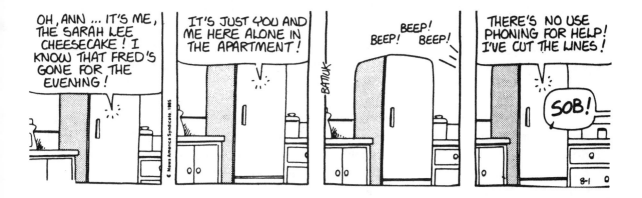

Our task in this lesson is to help you prevent lapses, but also to prevent lapses from becoming relapse, and finally to prevent relapse from becoming collapse.

Case Example.   Beth had lost 40 pounds and was working very hard to maintain the loss. During the 40-pound loss, she experienced only minor setbacks. She had learned to identify her eating triggers and managed to keep herself away from high-risk situations. She was exercising three times each week and was slowly gaining confidence that she would keep the weight off once and for all.

One day Beth drove to the convenience store to buy some milk, and on impulse decided to buy a bag of potato chips "for the kids." Vowing she would eat none herself, the bag called to her from the front seat of the car, so Beth opened it and took a few bites. By the time she got home, she had eaten quite a few chips.

When Beth entered the house, she was feeling guilty and ashamed. She had worked so hard to lose those 40 pounds that she could not believe she was slipping back into her old ways. She really liked the chips, however, and since she was feeling guilty anyway, she polished off the rest of the bag.

You can imagine what the bag of chips did to Beth's confidence. She thought about nothing else for the rest of the day, and the bloated feeling reminded her time and time again that she had failed herself. These feelings carried over to the next day and she began having fantasies about eating some of her favorite foods. She figured that since she had blown it, she may as well treat herself before she went back on her program.

She did treat herself, then treat herself again, and from there it was downhill. The good days were crowded out by the bad and Beth could not bring herself to get back on her program. As the lapses piled up, she finally gave up and concluded that she was hopeless.

Let's look at Beth as an example of how the lapse, relapse, and collapse terminology applies. Buying the chips, opening the bag in the car, feeling guilty, and eating the entire bag is a lapse. Beth could increase her chances of long-term maintenance by preventing lapses. So can you. You will be learning many techniques for preventing lapses, beginning with the process of risk assessment you read about in Chapter 3.

Beth's lapse created such negative feelings that she relapsed. She had more episodes of overeating and could not quite recover. After several weeks of relapsing, Beth collapsed. Before reading on, think of how Beth could have prevented the initial lapse from becoming relapse, and then even after she relapsed, how she could have prevented collapse. The information that follows will help you do this in your own life.

A Model of Lapse, Relapse, and Collapse

As different as people are from one another, lapse, relapse, and collapse usually proceed in an orderly way. Certain patterns emerge when we look at the thousands of dieters we have worked with and when we examine studies that have been done on this topic. We would like to spell out these patterns so you can see you are not alone, and can learn ways to apply this information to your weight maintenance plan.

Important work in this area has been done by two psychologists at the University of Washington, G. Alan Marlatt and Judith Gordon. They have studied lapse, relapse, and collapse in dieters, smokers, alcoholics, drug addicts, and compulsive gamblers. From this work, they developed a model for how and why relapse occurs. We have adapted this model to be specifically relevant for weight maintenance.

The figure you see in this section on the "Lapse and Relapse Process" shows how it all begins -- with a high-risk situation. In the case of Beth, buying a food she craved (potato chips) created a high-risk situation.

If you follow Path 1, at the top of the figure, you see what happens when dieters have learned coping skills. They use the skills. This increases their confidence they can handle risky situations, which leads to further control over eating.

Path 2 shows the course of someone who does not have the skills to handle the situation. The person lapses (initial eating). This undermines self-confidence, which can lead to further eating. If left unchecked, this leads to loss of control. Beth did not have the skills to stop after having a few potato chips. She saw her confidence slip away, and ultimately lost control.

Path 1 is certainly preferable to Path 2. The first step in making Path 1 a way-of-life is to recognize the different steps along the way. The two key aspects of Path 1 are skills and

The Process of Lapse and Relapse

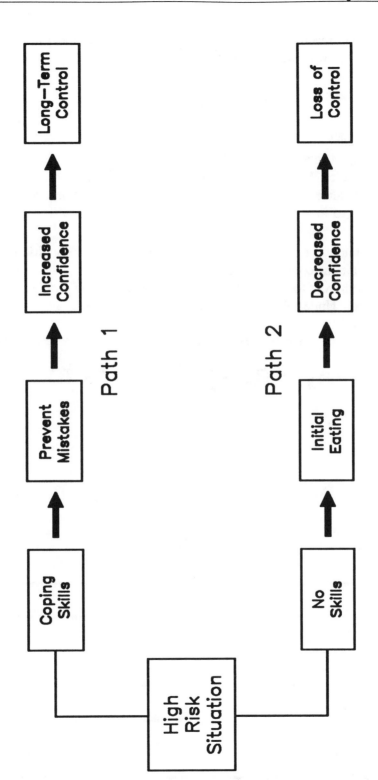

High Risk Situation

Coping Skills → Prevent Mistakes → Increased Confidence → Long-Term Control

Path 1

No Skills → Initial Eating → Decreased Confidence → Loss of Control

Path 2

Adapted from model in Relapse Prevention by Marlatt & Gordon (New York: Guilford, 1985).

confidence. We will teach you skills (both behaviors and attitudes) that will increase your confidence. Once you brim with confidence, the world is yours.

Back To Risk Assessment

Remember back to Chapter 3 (Risk Assessment). We described how to identify the situations, feelings, settings, moods, foods, and so forth that place you at risk. At that time, you completed a form called "My Eating Risk Factors." We have included a copy of that form in this lesson so you can complete it again now. You have now had more time to think about risk and to begin applying it to your own situation.

Take a few minutes to complete the form. Think about **any** conditions which create risk for you. List them in the column on the left and then note what creates the risk in the column on the right. If Beth were to fill this out, she would write "Having problem foods in the car" as one risky situation. Under What Creates Risk, she would have "alone, feeling hungry and deprived."

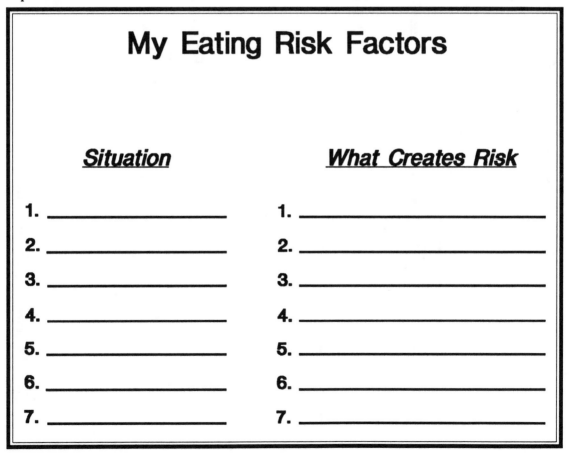

My Eating Risk Factors

Situation

1. _____
2. _____
3. _____
4. _____
5. _____
6. _____
7. _____

What Creates Risk

1. _____
2. _____
3. _____
4. _____
5. _____
6. _____
7. _____

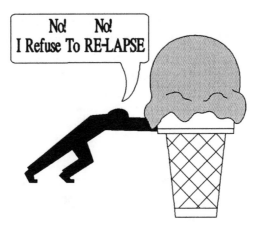

Now that you have a current list, we can forge ahead and develop plans for keeping on Path 1. You will be surprised by how much you can apply this to your life.

Preventing Lapses

A number of steps are available to you to prevent lapses. These begin with spotting danger and planning. This concept of being prepared will come up time and time again in this book.

Spotting Risk

One way to avoid trouble is to know where it lies. This is where the risk assessment discussed previously is so important. The goal is self-awareness. If you know when and where you will encounter risk, you can do something about it.

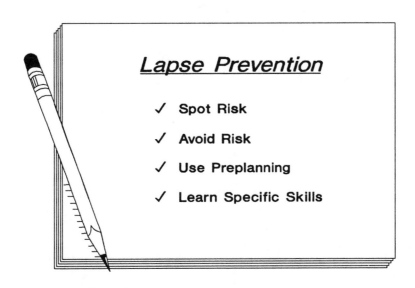

Think of the situations that put you at risk, using the risk factor list you completed earlier. What are the early warning signs? Almost all high-risk situations are preceded by warning signs. With Beth and the potato chips, it was feeling deprived, hungry, and weak that made her buy the chips once she went into the convenience store. If she had been sensitive to these feelings, she would have recognized that the situation was risky, and could have developed a preventive plan.

Avoiding Risk

If a situation will cause you trouble, the most straightforward remedy is to avoid the situation. In this case, an ounce of prevention is worth a pound of weight loss. This approach is practical in a surprising number of instances.

Let's say that driving past your favorite fast food restaurant is a set-up for temptation because the drive-in window tempts you like a worm tempts a fish. You could take another road that does not bring you by the window. If coming home from work in a crazed, hungry state is a problem, you could pack a salad and eat it just before you leave for home, or you could have a piece or two of fruit before you arrive. If having lunch alone weakens your resolve, try to have lunch with a friend.

These are just examples of how one person might avoid the risky situations. This is not possible all the time, of course, but whenever it **is** possible, do your best to stay out of trouble by avoiding trouble.

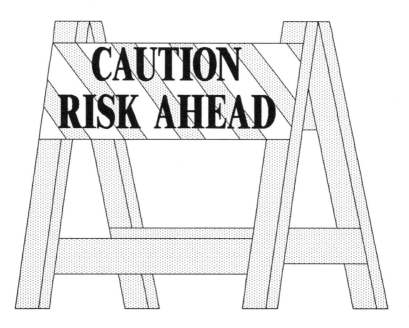

Preplanning

Do you know the Boy Scout Motto? It is to "Be Prepared." The rationale is that being prepared for any situation allows you to preplan. Then, even when you find yourself in a pickle, you will know what to do. If you are with the Scouts out in the woods, you must know what to do if confronted by bad weather, dangerous animals, or worst of all, Girl Scouts.

Here is another example of where preplanning is important. Think of fire drills in schools. Children are drilled time and time again, so when a real fire occurs, they will not panic and will leave the building in a safe, orderly way. It is critical that they know what to do in advance, so when danger occurs, no time is lost in making and executing a plan.

For weight maintenance, this preplanning philosophy is just as important. When confronted by temptation and in a weakened state, the mind is not always clear and logical. Rather than be surprised, have a plan for every situation you are likely to encounter. When in that situation, execute the plan just as the children execute the fire drill.

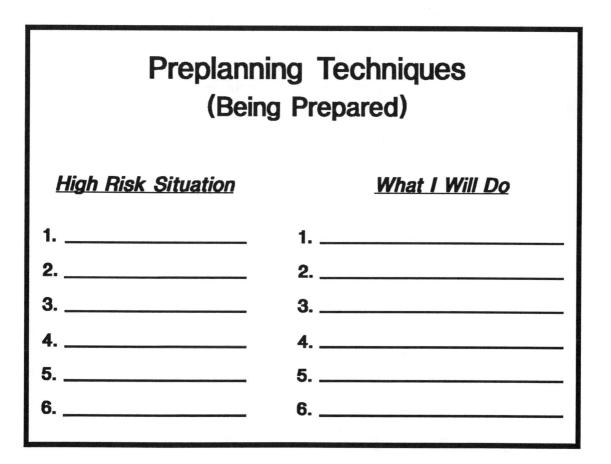

Preplanning Techniques
(Being Prepared)

High Risk Situation	_What I Will Do_
1. _____	1. _____
2. _____	2. _____
3. _____	3. _____
4. _____	4. _____
5. _____	5. _____
6. _____	6. _____

Use the chart on Preplanning Techniques to make your plans. Do it now so you are certain to complete the form. The high-risk situations can be taken from the risk factor form you completed earlier. Then write down what you will do when you are in that situation. Keep this plan handy and know in advance what you will do. This way you won't be surprised, you will be prepared.

Specific Skills

Learning specific skills will increase your confidence that you can master most situations. This way, you will not be fearful of temptations to eat and will be able to think in a clear and logical manner when trouble arises. An auto mechanic does not fear for his car breaking down because he has the skills to fix it. A comedian does not worry about a heckler in the audience because he or she knows how to handle the situation.

We will be working with you to develop specific ways to behave, think, and react if you lapse in your high-risk situations. If you can make a concrete plan, you will know **exactly** what to do when the right time comes. This will involve knowing the contexts in which you are at risk, and then knowing what to do when the conditions dictate.

Relapse Prevention

There are a number of ways to prevent lapses from turning to relapse. As you will see, there are both behaviors and attitudes that will pave the way for relapse prevention.

Relapse Prevention

✓ **Learn From Lapses**

✓ **React Constructively**

✓ **Avoid Catastrophic Reaction**

Learn From Lapse

Someone who does not learn from lapses is destined to repeat them (noted in 776 B.C by the ancient Greek dieter, Adiposites). Each time you stray from the path of your intended weight control, you have a valuable opportunity to learn. It is important to take advantage of each opportunity by analyzing the situation, deciding where you went wrong, and planning what can be done to prevent the lapse in the future. It is true that it is better to never lapse at all, but when one does, it is best to learn.

React Constructively

It is common for people to beat up on themselves emotionally when they make mistakes. In fact, some dieters say things to themselves they would not dream of saying to others. Examples are, "This proves I am worthless. I know I will be fat forever. I guess what others say is true -- I am a slob."

These internal thoughts can wear you down like the wind and rain wear away the topsoil. It is important to put these aside as soon as you recognize the negative feelings they create, and to react in a constructive way to all lapses.

Avoid Catastrophic Reactions

Another title for this section could be "Keeping Things In Perspective." Many people who are trying to control their weight overreact to even small mistakes. The consequence is bad feelings, which only distract them from learning and growing.

Even the worst eating binge is likely to add no more than 2 pounds of weight. Such a binge would derail most people because of their catastrophic reaction to losing control. Putting the weight gain in perspective, one might say "I wish I wouldn't have gained the weight, but the extra two pounds just means I'll have to bounce back again. I have done it before and this time I am determined to maintain." It is fine to note when you make mistakes and to be realistic about what you did wrong, but not to make yourself the victim of cruel and unusual punishment.

Using a Maintenance Road Map

Think of spreading out a road map before you. You can look at the map and locate trouble spots to avoid. This is the Risk Assessment we have discussed in such detail. You can then lay out what looks to be the safest and most uneventful course. However, you must be prepared for the worst.

Even the best planned trip will have detours. When you eat too much, fail to exercise, or lose control, you have taken a detour from your maintenance plan. If you are good with a map, you will pull it out, have confidence that you will find your way, and plot the most constructive course. This is where a cool head and the skills you have learned will be so valuable.

Think often of the road map example. You can use preplanning to plot your course, and remember that even if you get lost, you have only made a detour. You can still arrive in good shape at your final destination as long as you are confident and you know when to use the skills you have learned.

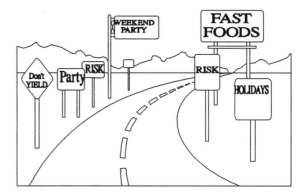

Watch For Signs Of High-Risk

Using a Maintenance Map

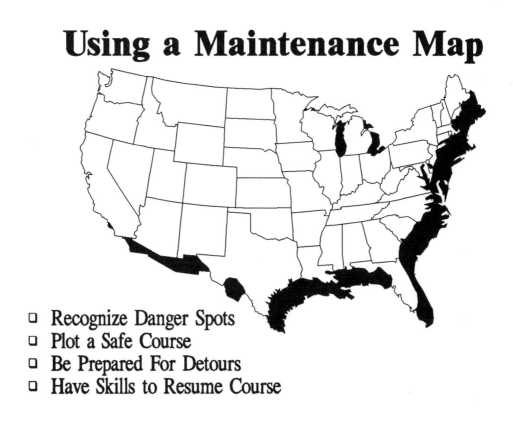

- ❑ Recognize Danger Spots
- ❑ Plot a Safe Course
- ❑ Be Prepared For Detours
- ❑ Have Skills to Resume Course

CHAPTER FIVE

Learning to Eat

Your Personal Computer

The human brain and nervous system is a natural computer. It has about two billion cells and can out-think and out-perform any artificial computer ever built. A great deal of programming is already in our computers when we are born. For example our heart, our lungs, our digestive systems and other vital functions run automatically. As we grow out of babyhood, our computers receive more and more programming: we learn to walk, talk, read, cook, fly a plane. Whatever we learn gets stored in our computers.

Your Eating Data Bank

We've also been programmed to eat. As infants, we learned that eating is a rewarding experience. If we cried, there was food and attention. We earned candy and ice cream by being good. This is how food and eating come to represent approval, as well as being a means for satisfying hunger. Is it surprising that adults turn to food to make themselves feel better?

We are also programmed to eat by external factors. The daily rhythm of our lives provides powerful cues to eat. As children we ate when the lunch bell rang, and after school we had a snack before going out to play. As adults we often eat because it has been scheduled into the day. We have coffee breaks, lunch meetings, dinner dates, etc.

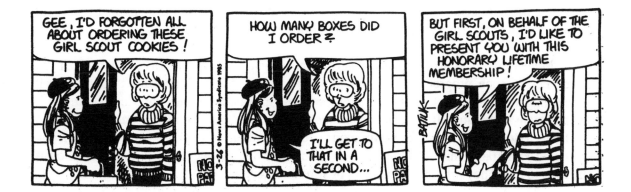

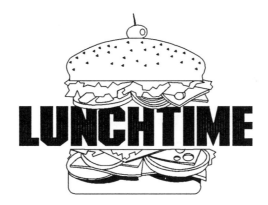

Time To Eat?

We associate eating with most social activities: going to a movie, watching a ball game, shopping, being with friends, and being part of nearly every holiday (Thanksgiving, Halloween, Valentines Day, etc.). Because we've all had these instructions built into our brains, they play an important role in determining when and how we eat.

These triggers must be identified for a person to lose weight, so you may have practiced some specific strategies already. For maintenance, we will show you the **principles** behind these strategies so that you can use the ones that work best for you.

Self Monitoring

Your 10,000 Mile Check Up

Remember the last time you went to the doctor for a check-up? You didn't think anything was wrong with you. It just seemed like a good time to check in and have a general once-over. You take care of your car the same way. This is a great maintenance strategy. You can use it for your eating behavior too. Every once-in-a-while it's time for that 10,000 mile check up, to be aware of the patterns in your behavior that influence your eating.

Many weight loss programs use a diary or monitoring form of one sort or another. If you have been in such programs, these are familiar to you. Most people don't continue self monitoring past the weight loss phase. Yet they feel guilty because they have learned that it is an important technique. It **is** an important technique, and should be used regularly while you are trying to **lose** weight. But for **maintenance**, food diaries are probably most useful when you are doing your 10,000 mile check-up. If you have never filled in such monitoring forms, now is the time to try. They will be helpful in all of your maintenance efforts.

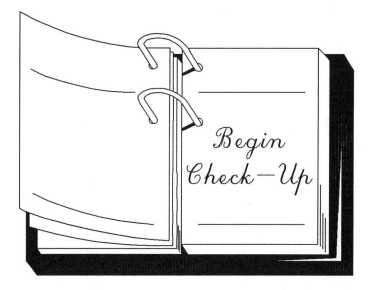

When Should You Monitor?

Some people use their diaries during maintenance at regular intervals; for example, once a month or once every six months. This is closer to the check-up idea. Other people use them when they have struggled with high-risk situations. You can tell **why** and **how** you are slipping by using these diaries, and by analyzing the problems. The purpose of the food diary is to reexamine your eating patterns.

Much of our eating is automatic. It occurs with little thought or attention. When you use a food diary, you are increasing your awareness.

What Should You Monitor?

What follows is an example of the kind of check-up monitor we recommend. This is a form completed by one of our clients, to show you how the form is used.

Following this sample form is a blank form for you to complete. Fill it out each time you eat and review seven day's worth at the end of each week so you can identify patterns.

We have provided a calorie guide in Appendix A that gives you calories for several hundred food items. If you need more information, there are calorie guides available in your supermarket or local bookstore. Most of them are based on a standard U.S. Department of Agriculture reference guide.

Food Diary

Food and Amount	Time	Feelings	Activity	Calories
BREAKFAST				
Coffee , 6 oz.	7:30	Tired	Paper	0
Scrambled Eggs, 2	"			222
Orange Juice , 1 cup	"			122
	TOTAL			344
LUNCH				
Roast Beef Sandwich	12:30	Hurried	Officework	241
Ritz Crackers , 6	"			90
Hot Cocoa , 1 cup	"			175
	TOTAL			506
DINNER				
Chicken Pot Pie	7:00	Relaxed	T.V.	545
Carrot-Raisin Salad	"			310
Cauliflower , 1 cup	"			28
Skim Milk , 1 cup	"			88
	TOTAL			971
SNACKS				
Candy Bar , 1½ oz.	2:45	Content	Reading Report	210
Coke , 12 oz.	3:15	Angry	Phone	144
Saltines , 5	9:15	Bored	T.V.	75
Peanut Butter, 2 tbsp.	"	"	"	188
	TOTAL			617

DAILY CALORIE TOTAL   2438

Food Diary

Food and Amount	Time	Feelings	Activity	Calories

BREAKFAST

_____	_____	_____	_____	_____
_____	_____	_____	_____	_____
_____	_____	_____	_____	_____
_____	_____	_____	_____	_____
	TOTAL			_____

LUNCH

_____	_____	_____	_____	_____
_____	_____	_____	_____	_____
_____	_____	_____	_____	_____
_____	_____	_____	_____	_____
	TOTAL			_____

DINNER

_____	_____	_____	_____	_____
_____	_____	_____	_____	_____
_____	_____	_____	_____	_____
	TOTAL			_____

SNACKS

_____	_____	_____	_____	_____
_____	_____	_____	_____	_____
_____	_____	_____	_____	_____
_____	_____	_____	_____	_____
	TOTAL			_____

DAILY CALORIE TOTAL _____

Searching For Patterns

Each week you will need to examine your food diaries for the past week and identify patterns. Here are some ideas for patterns to look for:

Foods   Pay close attention to the foods you eat. Are there patterns to the foods you choose? Which foods contribute most to your calories? Can you think of substitutes for the foods that have many calories? Are some foods more likely at certain times of day? If these are problem foods, can you think of substitute activities at that time?

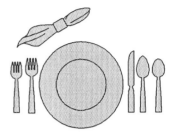

Amount   Look over the quantities and calories of the food you eat. One key is to enjoy the food you eat so there are no wasted calories. Are there foods you could eat less of or avoid completely? Do you eat specific amounts each time, without thinking about how much you need and want?

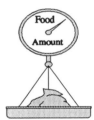

Time   Look for times of the day when you are likely to eat. A typical pattern shows little eating at breakfast and lunch, but much eating and snacking at dinner and after. Try to spread your calories out more through the day. Do you crave a snack just before bed? Do you always have something in mid-afternoon? Are your meals irregular? Do you skip meals? Again, a more spread-out pattern may work better for you.

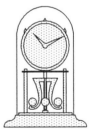

Feelings   Do you eat when you are bored, depressed, anxious, angry, or lonely? Other feelings may also be involved, like resentment, hostility, jealousy, or even joy. Seeing a pattern is a sure sign that you can learn more adaptive ways to cope with difficult feelings.

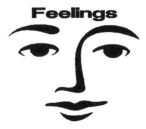

Activity   What do you do while eating? Watching television is the main culprit, but reading a newspaper, listening to a radio, or browsing through magazines can also be a problem. Doing two things at once insures that neither gets full attention. Eating gets less attention than it deserves. Eating should be separated from other activities.

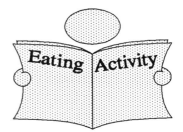

Calories   If you are within 10-15 calories for each item, your calorie awareness is high. If you underestimate most foods, however, study the calorie guide.

When you analyze your check-up monitors, be careful not to evaluate yourself too harshly. Don't demand perfect eating habits of yourself -- that's like pursuing Don Quixote's "Impossible Dream." Look instead for the places where you might be slipping away from your newly acquired habits. When you find that you've slipped, apply the strategies you've learned to reinstate and reinforce your good habits.

Be realistic in your self-analysis. Did you set your goals too high? Revise them to make them reachable. On the other hand, if your analysis showed you had everything under control, you may not be looking hard enough at yourself.

When Should You Stop?

How will you know when your check-up is over? Monitoring during maintenance is to provide you with information. You are ready to stop when you have mastered two important points.

First, you need to be able to identify your patterns. You can stop when you feel comfortable that you know **what** and **how much** you are eating, the **times** of day that you eat, the **moods** and **feelings** that make you eat, and the **places** and **activities** associated with eating.

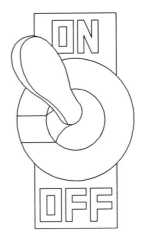

You are also ready to stop when you can estimate how many calories you've eaten each day. When you feel confident that you can correctly count the calories you've eaten by simply reviewing the foods that you had that day, continual monitoring may not be necessary.

When To Stop?

After you have stopped recording in your diaries, think about your patterns for that day at night, before you go to bed. If you feel confident that you can clearly say what you did that day, review your patterns for the whole week in your mind. Here you need to think about generalities, rather then specifics. On the average, are there good and bad times of day? On the average, does feeling sad make you eat more than feeling angry? When you are confident that you can identify your patterns correctly, your check-up is over for this period. Good work!

Evaluating Your Patterns

Most good weight loss programs emphasize some helpful behavioral patterns. The table on the next page summarizes the kinds of advice that such weight loss programs include.

While all of these principles are helpful for weight loss, you may use them more flexibly for weight maintenance. Some of them are too restrictive, others too artificial. Only some can be incorporated into your particular lifestyle.

For maintenance, you must set your own guidelines, and use them consistently. One person might say, "I am not going to do anything else while eating. I will eat all my food in the same place and I will always leave some food on the plate." Another person's guidelines might include leaving the table immediately after eating, chewing thoroughly, and avoiding ready-to-eat foods. The next chapter will help you choose your own lifestyle guidelines for successful maintenance.

A Check-Up Schedule Preview

We will come back to this idea of regular check-ups in Chapter 12. There we will outline a specific maintenance schedule for using the quizzes and monitoring forms that are introduced in earlier chapters. One of these will be the food diary. By doing regular assessments of your eating, attitudes, and other important factors, you will be able to spot trouble in early stages. Then you can use the skills you have learned to return to the right track.

When we discuss regular check-ups in Chapter 12, we will discuss the importance of early warning signs. Every three months, you will have several questionnaires and quizzes to complete. Depending on your answers, we will help you know how to proceed with your maintenance plan. This way, you can strike the right balance between being alert and thinking too much about eating and weight.

To help with these regular check-ups, we have developed a Maintenance Kit that contains the necessary forms and a check-up schedule. This can be ordered using the information provided at the end of this book.

<u>Tips for Behavioral Control of Eating</u>

<u>Shopping</u>

- Shop for food after eating (i.e., when not physically hungry)
- Shop from a prepared list
- Avoid ready-to-eat foods
- Don't carry more cash than needed for shopping list

<u>Plans</u>

- Plan in advance to limit food intake in a particular way
- Eat meals and snacks at scheduled times

<u>Activities</u>

- Store food out of sight
- Remove food from places other than kitchen or dining room (e.g. bedroom, desk at work, car)
- Eat only in kitchen or dining room
- Keep serving dishes off the table
- Use smaller dishes and serving utensils
- Leave the table immediately after eating
- Have other people clean up the dishes
- Don't save high-calorie leftovers
- Don't participate in other activities while eating (e.g., reading, watching TV)
- Don't clean your plate
- Put your fork down sometimes between bites

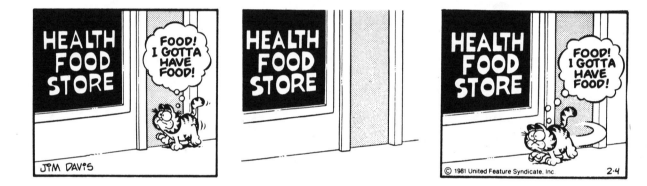

CHAPTER SIX

Charting Your Course

Your Lifestyle Guidelines

We have been emphasizing how maintenance is different from the times when you are trying to lose weight. Maintenance is for the rest of your life. It can't feel like a diet and work well.

We now move to an important matter -- how to set guidelines for maintenance. They will be based on what you learned from your check-up monitors in the last chapter. They also depend on your own insights about what you believe you can do in a sustained way. Just like setting a realistic weight goal, you need to have realistic expectations for what will and won't work, given your own, unique life. These expectations will be your signposts for success.

Your Calorie Guidelines

What about calories? You can develop many helpful strategies when your caloric awareness is high.

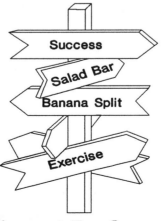

Signpost For Success

Maintain Calorie Range

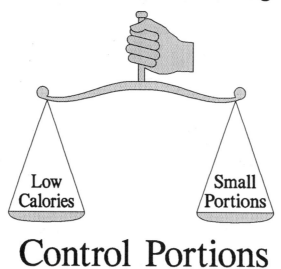

Low
Calories

Small
Portions

Control Portions

You may no longer need to measure the amount of food you are consuming, if you know calories well enough to guide yourself within an acceptable margin of error. If you eat too many calories on one day, you can restrict your caloric intake gradually over the next few days. If you cut down too drastically, you may slow down your metabolism.

Try substituting low-calorie alternatives for higher-calorie foods, for example, ice milk or low-fat yogurt vs. ice cream, rather than cutting out foods entirely. You can also reduce the **amount** of food you eat, rather than changing the **type** of food you eat. This is especially important in making decisions about foods you eat in their natural state. For example, we tend to think of fruits as non-fattening foods. Yet fruits vary enormously in size. Smaller pieces of fruit contain fewer calories. Portion control is a great way to cut down without cutting out.

Include some calorie strategies on the "guidelines" chart you will be completing later in this chapter. They should be ones that can realistically work for you. One recommendation though. Set a **range** of calories that is acceptable to you on a daily basis rather than a specific target number. It is impossible for any of us to keep to a specific set of calories without falling prey to the diet mentality.

How Do You Eat?

Most Americans eat three meals a day. Our school and work schedules are arranged that way, and most of our daily activities revolve around this kind of meal pattern. But some of us are different. We don't work or go to school. Our families don't come home for dinner or start the morning together. So, recommending three meals a day is not part of this program. In fact, one recent study found that people eating many small meals during the day had a more favorable physiological response than did people eating the same number of calories in three meals.

The body is fired up every time you eat. Some calories are burned by the work your body needs to do to digest the food you eat. If you prefer eating frequent small meals, rather than three large meals, and this works for your life style, you might want to try this strategy.

Some of you eat just one or two meals a day. The scientific evidence shows that eating at least three meals a day is essential. Too many people who are overweight tend to eat nothing all day and then begin to eat at dinner and continue late into the evening. Not only is this a bad strategy in terms of metabolism, but night time eating is typically where most people get into trouble.

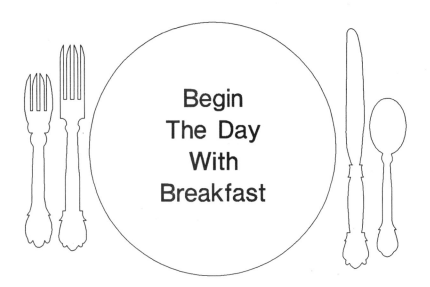

Start with a good breakfast. Breakfast is important because it gets your metabolism going after it has slowed down during the night. Even if your breakfast is small, this metabolic kick off is important for a good day. Notice that we are not saying what to eat. Just eat **something** as you start your day. Many overweight people eat no breakfast when they are gaining weight, and then begin to eat breakfast as they lose.

Binging, Sneaking and Grazing

Are you a binge eater? This is a problem for some people who are trying to maintain their weight. Answer the questions on the following page to see.

Eating Habits Checklist

Instructions. Below are groups of numbered statements. Read all of the statements in each group and mark the one that best describes the way you feel about the problems you have controlling your eating behavior.

#1

(0)   1.   I don't have any difficulty eating slowly in the proper manner.

(1)   2.   Although I seem to "gobble down" foods, I don't end up feeling stuffed because of eating too much.

(2)   3.   At times, I tend to eat quickly and then, I feel uncomfortably full afterwards.

(3)   4.   I have the habit of bolting down my food, without really chewing it. When this happens I usually feel uncomfortably stuffed because I've eaten too much.

#2

(0)   1.   I feel capable to control my eating urges when I want to.

(1)   2.   I feel like I have failed to control my eating more than the average person.

(3)   3.   I feel utterly helpless when it comes to feeling in control of my eating urges.

(3)   4.   Because I feel so helpless about controlling my eating I have become very desperate about trying to get in control.

#3

(0)   1.   I don't lose total control of my eating when dieting even after periods when I overeat.

(2)   2.   Sometimes when I eat a "forbidden food" on a diet, I feel like I "blew it" and eat even more.

(3)   3.   Frequently, I have the habit of saying to myself, "I've blown it now, why not go all the way" when I overeat on a diet. When that happens I eat even more.

(3)   4.   I have a regular habit of starting strict diets for myself, but I break the diets by going on an eating binge. My life seems to be either a "feast" or "famine."

Eating Habits Checklist (continued)

#4

(0)   1.   I usually am able to stop eating when I want to. I know when "enough is enough."

(1)   2.   Every so often, I experience a compulsion to eat which I can't seem to control.

(2)   3.   Frequently, I experience strong urges to eat which I seem unable to control, but at other times I can control my eating urges.

(3)   4.   I feel incapable of controlling urges to eat. I have a fear of not being able to stop eating voluntarily.

#5.

(0)   1.   I don't think about food a great deal.

(1)   2.   I have strong cravings for food but they last only for brief periods of time.

(2)   3.   I have days when I can't seem to think about anything else but food.

(3)   4.   Most of my days seem to be preoccupied with thoughts about food. I feel like I live to eat.

The scoring weights are in parentheses next to each statement. Your total score is the sum of the weights of the items you checked for the set of 5 statements. The higher your score, the more of a binge eater you are.

This scale was adapted from The Eating Habits Check List, by James Gormally, Ph.D. Used with permission.

The Binger

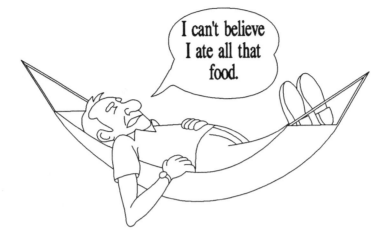

Bingers are people filled with good intentions. They set off to be a "good dieter," which is sometimes successful, at least temporarily. Then the restriction becomes too much and a binge breaks through.

When bingers fall off the wagon they do it with style. Often people binge because they feel both guilty and deprived. There is no such thing as wrong foods or right foods in weight maintenance, so there is nothing to feel guilty about. You can have the foods you like. You simply need to have them less often or have them in smaller amounts. You are more likely to binge when you tell yourself you shouldn't be having what you're eating.

The Sneaker

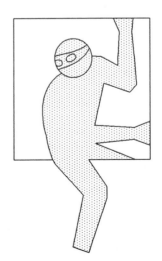

Other people are sneakers.

Sneakers are the people who eat nothing in public and then at home, stuff themselves in secret. Sneakers hide candy bars in the bathroom or under the bed. They never eat at parties since they don't want the outside world to see their weaknesses. Successful maintainers are those who find foods that they are willing to eat in public, as well as in private. If you have private or secret foods, an important task for successful maintenance is to eat them in public. Don't keep secrets when it comes to food.

The Grazer

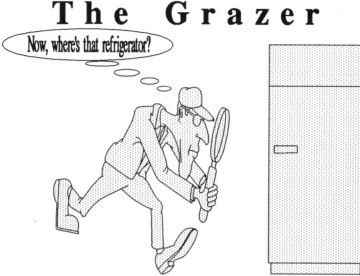

Now, where's that refrigerator?

Some people are grazers. **Grazers** are people who spend a lot of time "window-shopping" at the refrigerator. They are always eating -- a little here and a little there, as if small pieces don't add up to large amounts. Some grazers never eat a reasonable-sized portion at one time so they never feel really satisfied. Long-term maintenance depends on feeling satisfied.

ARE YOU A

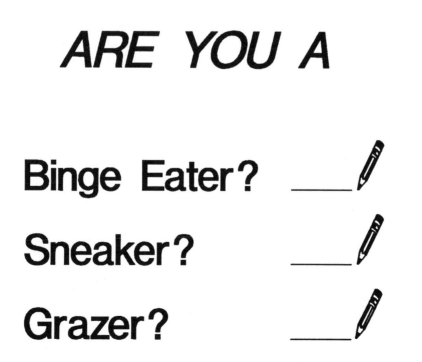

Binge Eater? _____

Sneaker? _____

Grazer? _____

Cut Down, Not Out

A key to successful maintenance is avoiding periods of deprivation. Lots of people who have trouble controlling their weight are restrained eaters. They give much thought and attention to food, and are always restraining what they eat, how much they eat, or when they eat.

Research shows that restrained eating leads to problems. For example, in some studies restrained eaters are given either a large milkshake to drink as part of a taste test, or no milkshake. Then they are all given a large bowl of ice cream and encouraged to eat as much as they need to rate the taste of the ice cream along several dimensions. The restrained eaters eat much more ice cream if they first had the milkshake than if they had nothing. Rather than seeming full from the milkshake, people who are restrained eaters overeat when they have already eaten what they think is too much. It's as if they feel, "what's the difference? I already ruined it for today, so I might as well have everything I've been missing and get back on the wagon tomorrow." This is a part of the diet mentality that doesn't work for maintenance.

How you eat is up to you, but maintenance depends on finding a set of guidelines that allow you to give **less, not more** conscious thought and attention to restricting your intake.

Cut Down, Not Out

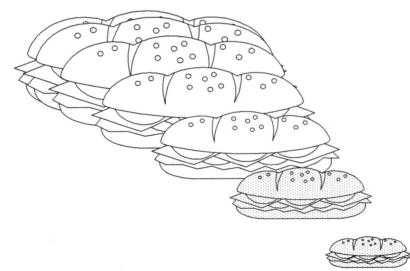

Achieving Structured Flexibility

Your Lifestyle Guidelines.

It is crucial to set guidelines that **you** can use. Think of them as lifestyle changes, rather than weight control strategies. Don't use strategies that are artificial for you because it is too hard to keep them going, but do develop a set of guidelines. When you can use your guidelines at least every day or more, you are on the-road to maintenance.

My Lifestyle Technique Guidelines are:

Avoid eating after 10:00 PM.

Exercise between 2 and 4 times each week.

Have between 400 and 600 calories for dinner.

Spend 10 minutes on Saturday morning reviewing my week
  and planning the changes I can make for next week, if any.

Below is a chart for you to fill in for your own lifestyle guidelines. They should help you to break the problem patterns you identified in your 10,000 mile check-up. We've provided a few examples of what other people have selected, but there are no "right" answers here.

My Lifestyle Technique Guidelines are:

Blueprint for Success

Remember that you want to learn the reasons behind the strategies, not just the strategies themselves. Now you are ready. Learning to eat for maintenance depends on three general principles.

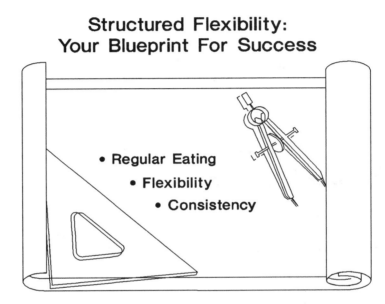

Structured Flexibility:
Your Blueprint For Success

- Regular Eating
- Flexibility
- Consistency

First, you need to throw away irregular eating. People who eat chaotically, without plans or guidelines, get into trouble. Plans and guidelines, which you set yourself, are your tools. They help you steer a clear course, around the obstacles and in stormy weather.

Second, your guidelines need flexibility as well as structure. Your guidelines have to be flexible enough so that you don't feel like you're on a diet. For example, yours may be to eat three meals a day or to eat only while you are hungry, but you need to have flexibility. If your friends take you out for brunch, eat a "breakfast-sized" amount. You can still eat a small second meal later in the day.

Third, you need to develop consistency. No matter what your guidelines are, you need to follow them consistently. When you deviate, do so only within your plan of structured flexibility. If you cannot be consistent, it's time to go back for a check-up and redo your food diaries.

In looking ahead to long-term maintenance, don't think of your guidelines as regulations or obligations. Instead, use them positively to keep yourself on track.

Long-Term Maintenance

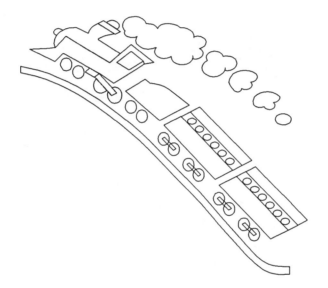

Keeping On Track

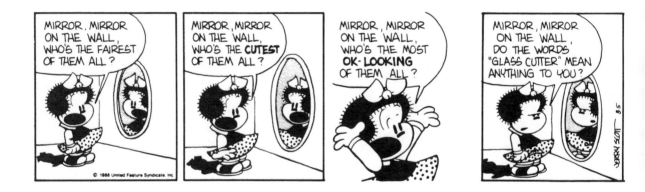

CHAPTER SEVEN

Exercise: Your Ticket To Long-Term Success?

Just How Important Is It?

Everybody knows that exercise is important, right? We see it in magazine and newspaper articles, and every expert on weight loss is quick to mention that a program should combine a good diet, behavior change, and yes, exercise.

Unfortunately, many people greet this realization with a sinking feeling. They feel they must get up at the crack of dawn to do the "Morning Stretch" with Miss Goodbody. Or, they must be working out in trendy clothing and accessories (like leg warmers). Neither is necessarily true. We believe that exercise can be a **big** help, but you may be surprised at the way we approach it.

Exercise and Long-Term Weight Control

Exercise is one of the few factors that distinguishes people who maintain weight loss from those who do not. We say this without reservation.

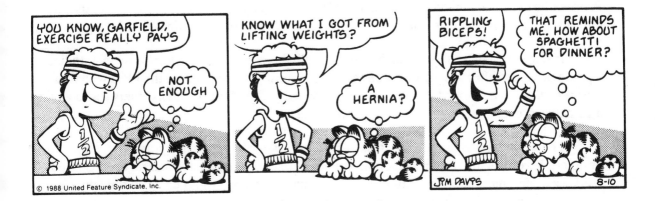

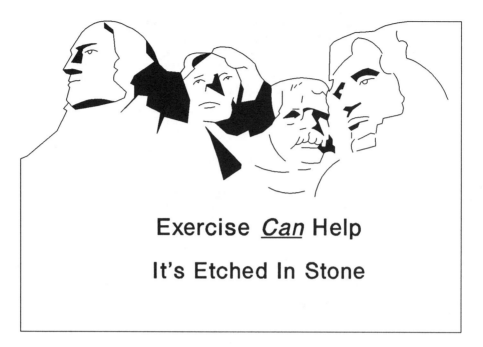

Exercise _Can_ Help

It's Etched In Stone

This may surprise you because you may know people (perhaps you are one yourself), who have lost weight without doing a lick of exercise. In fact, one of our successful patients once said, "When I get the urge to exercise, I lie down until it goes away."

How do we reconcile stories like these with the fact that people who exercise are most likely to keep their weight off? Part of the answer lies in the way the issue has been studied by scientists. Two approaches have been used to examine exercise and weight loss.

The first method is to follow people some time after a weight loss program has ended. People who have maintained can be compared to those who have regained to see what they do differently. In such studies, the maintainers are more likely to be exercising than the regainers.

In one such a study, Drs. Susan Kayman, Judith Stern and colleagues in California studied a group of women after weight loss. They compared those who maintained their loss with those who regained. When asked, "Do you exercise regularly?," 92% of the maintainers responded affirmatively, compared to only 34% of the regainers.

The second way to study exercise is to randomly assign people to programs that either do or do not have structured exercise. Some studies have compared exercise to no exercise from the very beginning, while other studies have compared exercise to no exercise only during a maintenance phase. Using both approaches, groups following the exercise program do better.

One interesting finding from these studies is that people who exercise typically do not lose more in the initial phases of a program (the first 3 or 4 months), but they **do** lose more in the long-run. Therefore, there seems to be something special about exercise and the **maintenance** of weight loss. This is why the topic deserves great emphasis in a book on maintaining weight loss.

Why It Is Important: Let Us Count The Ways

If we walk down the street and ask the first 100 people we meet why exercise is important for weight loss, the majority will answer "Because it burns calories." They are only partially right.

Exercise does burn calories, but probably not as many as you think. For example, a person who goes to McDonald's for lunch and has a Big Mac, small fries, and chocolate shake, has just eaten 1,173 calories. Do you know how many miles someone must jog to burn off those calories? Since you burn about 100 calories per mile, one must jog 11.73 miles to burn off the calories in that single meal.

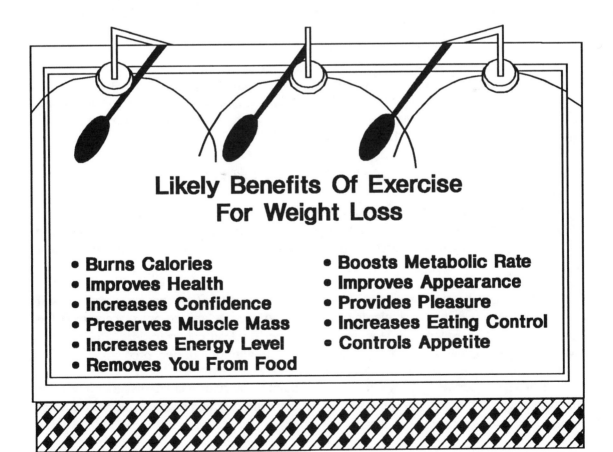

Likely Benefits Of Exercise For Weight Loss

- Burns Calories
- Improves Health
- Increases Confidence
- Preserves Muscle Mass
- Increases Energy Level
- Removes You From Food
- Boosts Metabolic Rate
- Improves Appearance
- Provides Pleasure
- Increases Eating Control
- Controls Appetite

One mistake many people make is to despair at figures like these and feel that exercise is fruitless. Others make the opposite mistake by feeling that because they exercise, they can afford to eat more, and they ultimately overdo it.

The calorie-burning value of exercise **can** be substantial. It is important, however, to focus not only on this virtue of exercise but on the other benefits as well.

Why Does Exercise Help?

The figure on the previous page lists some of the ways exercise is thought to aid in weight loss. We say "thought to aid" because some points are better documented than others. For instance, in studies of metabolism in non-overweight people, exercise does boost metabolic rate. What it does in people who are dieting has not been studied in sufficient detail to proclaim its impact.

Another example is the food intake issue. There are animal studies, and some data in humans, that exercise helps the individual regulate weight at a normal level, even in the presence of a diet that would otherwise lead to obesity. A study with rats by Dr. Judith Stern and colleagues found that animals that went on and off high-fat diets developed a greater preference for fat in the diet. Exercise prevented this.

There is a detailed scientific literature on exercise and body weight. From our analysis of the evidence, we feel that one thing is clear -- exercise is associated with long-term success. Whether it does so for psychological or physiological reasons is not known, but one might well say, "So what? As long as it works, I'm going to give it a try."

Beware of the Negative Expectation

It may sound from the previous discussion that we are exercise crusaders. This is true of many experts on weight control. The positive side of this crusade is that more people begin to think that exercise may help keep weight off. The negative side is that some people believe that exercise is **the** key to success.

Do **not** feel that exercise is the only way to keep weight off, or that you are doomed if you do not exercise. There are plenty of people who exercise and do not succeed over the long-run and there are plenty who lose weight and keep it off with no exercise. Stated another way, exercise is associated with weight maintenance, but it is not a perfect predictor.

You might be asking why we bring up this point. The reason is that we do not want to plant the idea that people who can't or won't exercise are destined to fail. This notion is not

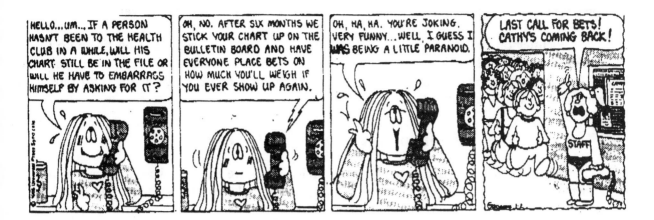

justified by our experience or the studies. We know that some of you will exercise and some will not. Those who will not should still feel confident they can lose weight and keep it off.

We do hasten to add that exercise may be one of the most valuable things you can do. We urge **all** people to learn the benefits of exercise, to understand its value in long-term weight control, and to give it a valid try before deciding it is not for them.

We perceive exercise as a valuable resource, much like a precious mineral lying beneath the ground. The resource is there for the taking, but diligence, persistence, and hard work are necessary to exploit it.

It is crucial to remember one point. You will never know whether a **good** exercise program will be right for you until you give it a try. Just because you have tried exercise before and have given it up does not mean that **our** approach cannot work for you. This approach is different from others you have tried. So, even if you are skeptical about whether exercise is for you, read on!

Consistency Vs. Type of Exercise

One question we are always asked at lectures is "What type of exercise should I do?" One interesting finding from exercise studies is that consistency seems more important than the type of exercise. In other words, doing something regularly may be as important as what you do.

This is one area where our advice might run contrary to what you have heard elsewhere. Many people believe there is only one "right" type of exercise, but as we will explain shortly, what is right depends on what you hope to accomplish. Aerobics is not necessarily better than some other type of activity, if we accept the proposition that consistency is the key.

Focusing on consistency raises a whole new set of questions, such as "How much do I enjoy a certain type of exercise?" or "What am I able to build into my routine?" As you will soon see, these questions may be more important to the dieter than questions about heart rate, coronary efficiency, and so forth.

The Trap of An Exercise Threshold

In addition to being asked what type of exercise is best, we are also asked, "How much do I have to do?" It is common for dieters to exercise, but to feel they have accomplished little.

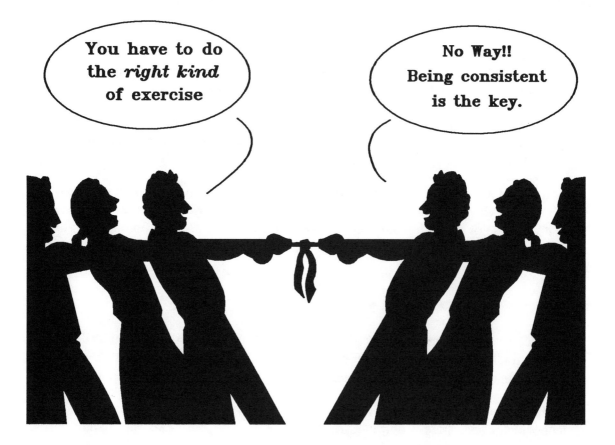

Here is how this happens. Deep in the psyche of most people is the notion that you have to do a lot of exercise to benefit. This comes from several sources. The first is the old-time mentality of coaches and gym teachers. They communicated the "No Pain, No Gain" philosophy. An entire generation was raised with the feeling that if you sweated and strained to within an inch of your life, you had a successful bout of exercise.

The second source comes from research on exercise and performance on exercise tests (like a treadmill or bicycle ergometer test). Doing careful research, scientists have found that to improve performance on such a test , one must have a combination of three things: frequency, intensity, and duration.

These three things **are** important if your aim is to improve your performance on the treadmill or bicycle, but this is not the only reason you want to exercise. You want to feel better, look better, and have more strength to stay with your weight maintenance plan. To accomplish these, frequency may be important (consistency), but having the right combination of this with intensity and duration may be less so.

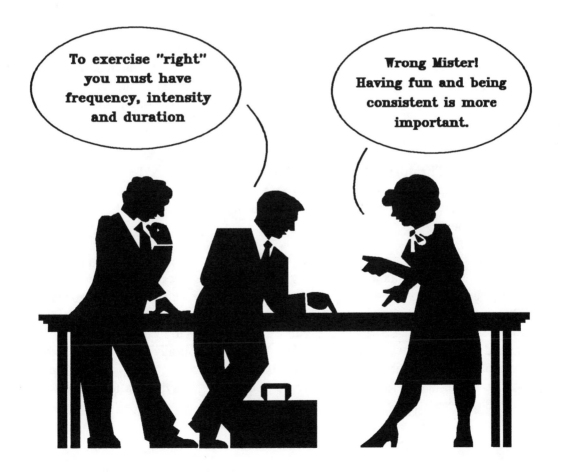

For your information, the exercise equation contains the following specifics:

Frequency. You must exercise at least 3 times per week.

Intensity. Your heart rate must increase to 70% or more of its maximum level. The maximum level can be estimated by subtracting your age from 220. For example, maximum heart rate for a 40-year-old would be 180, and for a 30-year-old would be 190. Calculate 70% of your maximum heart rate, and this is where your heart rate should be during exercise.

Duration. During each bout of exercise, your heart rate should stay in this zone for at least 20 minutes.

This information **is** important when you want to improve your fitness level. However, you can put this on the back burner until you are able to integrate exercise into your life and make some form of activity **consistent** in your day-to-day routine.

The Health Benefits of Modest Activity

Two studies show that you don't have to be a triathlete to obtain health benefits from exercise. Dr. Steven Blair and colleagues at the Institute of Aerobics Research in Dallas studied physical fitness and health in more than 13,000 men and women. These individuals had been given detailed medical exams, and were then followed for an average of eight years. One part of the exam was a stress test on a treadmill to measure physical fitness.

The Blair study found striking health benefits for people who were just moderately fit. On the main index of health used by the researchers, risk was reduced by half for people with a "moderate" level of fitness, compared to those who were least fit. Blair and associates concluded that a regular walking program could move a person from the least fit to the moderately fit group.

Another study, this one by Dr. James Rippe and colleagues at the University of Massachusetts Medical Center, looked at walking and weight loss. People who dieted without a walking program lost an average of 17 pounds, but 25% of their weight loss was lean body mass (muscle). People who combined the diet with a walking program also lost 17 pounds, but only 6% of the loss was muscle. The goal in weight loss, of course, is to lose fat. One advantage of losing fat and preserving muscle is that muscle is more metabolically active than fat, so more calories are burned to sustain muscle than the same amount of fat. The people in this study were not followed for a long time, but if they were, we would guess that **maintenance** would be better for the walkers.

How To Do Exercise Right

The trick to picking the "right" type of exercise is to ask yourself the right questions. Some of these questions are in the Exercise Quiz. Take the quiz and sketch out your answers. You can then use your responses to make exercise right for you.

Exercise Quiz

1. **Do you prefer to exercise alone or with others?**   _____

2. **Does your climate permit regular outdoor exercise?**   _____

3. **Are you embarassed to be seen while exercising?**   _____

4. **Do you prefer a place to go to exercise (like a club)?**   _____

5. **Do you prefer an instructor to lead you?**   _____

6. **Will you exercise regularly at home?**   _____

7. **Are you willing to work exercise into your routine?**   _____

8. **What is your favorite way to be active?**   _____

9. **Would you prefer to do different things on different days, or do the same thing all the time?**   _____

You can probably tell where we are heading. We obviously have a liberal definition of exercise and realize that different activities will be right for different people. Therefore, the world holds open a vast array of exercise possibilities. Things you previously thought didn't "count," like bowling, golf, leisurely walks, and gardening, do count if they work for you.

The important thing is to define yourself as being physically active. If you consider yourself an exerciser, the label will mean a lot and will help you in every aspect of weight maintenance. This is why consistency is more important than the type of exercise. Each time you exercise, no matter how you do it, you are sending a signal to your self-esteem that you are making positive changes. This will increase your self-confidence and propel you on your way.

In picking an exercise, think of the following issues:

1)   **Is It Fun?** If you like it, you'll do it. If you hate it, you're asking for grief. Above all, exercise should be fun. Please remember that it **can** be fun. It can be a nice social event, you can explore the countryside, you can meet new people, and you can feel good about yourself and your body.

2)   **Will You Do It Regularly?** Doing something once or twice won't be much help, so ask yourself if you can envision doing something on a consistent basis. The things to consider are how it fits with your work and family schedule, whether it is reasonable given where you live, whether it can fit practically into the time you can set aside, and whether you feel you would enjoy it as you do it over the upcoming weeks and months.

Selecting An Activity Program

All the talk up to this point is aimed in one direction -- helping you pick an activity or activities that will become part of your routine. Once we do this, you will need to experiment and fine-tune your program until it suits your lifestyle.

The accompanying figure shows a list of activities. These are examples of the things you might select. Start by going through the list and checking everything you might enjoy. Then go back over the ones you have picked and narrow the list to those you are pretty certain you would enjoy and would consider doing, at least once in awhile.

Next, think of how you might schedule the one or more activities you picked. Remember, it is certainly fine to do different things in your program. You might play tennis with a friend once each week, ride the exercise bike during a few favorite TV shows, and then walk by yourself or with a friend one or two times each week. As long as you do **something** consistently, you are moving in the right direction.

Programmed Activities

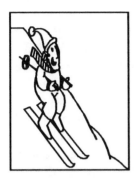

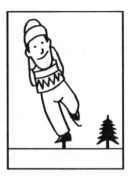

Aerobics

Badminton

Bowling

Calisthenics

Cycling

Dancing

Golf

Handball

Hiking

Horseback

Jogging

Mall Walking

Nautilus

Racquetball

Skating

Skiing

Slimnastics

Softball

Squash

Swimming

Tennis

Video

Walking

Weights

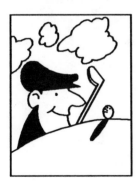

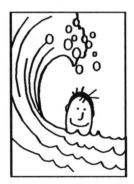

Is Walking The Answer?

For many people, walking **is** the answer. It can lead to significant health benefits, can help with weight control, and can make you feel good. It is available to almost everyone, and can be done in different times and in different places. It can be done fast or slow, and can be done by yourself or with others. There are walking shoes, walking clothes, walking clubs, walking books, walking magazines, and before long, we might even have a "walker's high!" People walk in malls, up and down stairs, in the hallways of buildings, and in many creative locations.

A number of resources are available for the person who walks. If you want company, call the nearest malls and ask if people walk there in the mornings. Go and talk to the walkers to see if there is an organized group or club. Even if this is not the case, you will meet people who are like you. Call the nearest YMCA or YWCA and ask if they sponsor walking groups. If they do not, the staff will likely know of other groups in your area. Finally, if you are a born leader, you can always organize your own group.

There are also national resources available. The list shown on the opposite page gives addresses of groups who can provide you with information on walking, including pamphlets, schedules of organized walks, and subscriptions to walking newsletters and magazines.

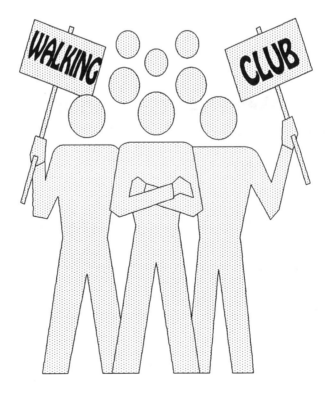

Resources for Walkers

American Volksport Association
1001 Pat Booker Road, Suite 203
Universal City, TX 78148
512-659-2112

Can send you a list of walking clubs in your area. Publishes *American Wanderer* $12 per yr. subscription ($8 bulk rate).

Prevention Walking Club
Rodale Press
Box 6099
Emmaus, PA 18099
800-441-7761

Quarterly newsletter and annual magazine dealing with all aspects of walking.
Membership cost is $9.97 per year

Rockport Walking Institute
P.O. Box 480
Marlboro, MA 01752
508-485-2090 (ext. 114)

Will send educational materials on fitness walking, diet and exercise. Call or send self-addressed business-sized envelope with $.45 postage affixed.

Walkabout International
835 Fifth Avenue, Room 407
San Diego, CA 92101

Club with chapters in various cities. Organizes & publishes information about walks.

WalkWays Center
733 15th Street, NW
Washington, D.C. 20005
202-737-9555

Non-profit clearing house for information on aspects of walking. Publishes a newsletter (*WalkWays Almanac*) 8 times per year; $17 for 1 year, $29 for 2 years.

Walking Magazine
Raben Publishing
711 Boylston Street
Boston, MA 02116
617-236-1885

Bi monthly commercial magazine about walking. $12 per yr. for subscription.

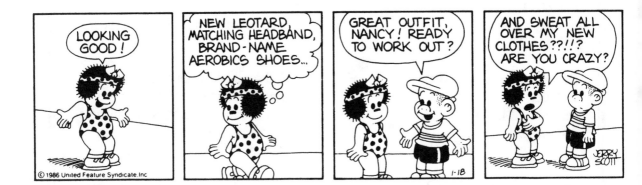

CHAPTER EIGHT

Eating Smart and Eating Right

Is Nutrition Important For Weight Maintenance?

Yes. Nutrition **is** important for weight maintenance, perhaps even more so than for weight loss.

Why? Because maintenance is helping to establish a permanent, more healthy lifestyle, and because what you eat influences how you think and how you feel. It is a mistake to feel that nutrition is a simple matter that can be overlooked.

We all know that nutrition is related to health. This is why many people are watching their intake of saturated fat and cholesterol, increasing fiber, and limiting salt. Even if good nutrition did not help you maintain your weight loss, which it will, it would make sense to eat the right foods for better health.

How sensitive our nation is about nutrition news is evident from the craze about oat bran. Based on the results of one small study, the media made oat bran newsworthy by declaring that it lowers cholesterol. The food companies were quick to exploit this by adding oats to various foods, including potato chips and beer! The money rolled in. One of the leading cereal companies was said to lose millions of dollars because they were too late onto the oat bran bandwagon.

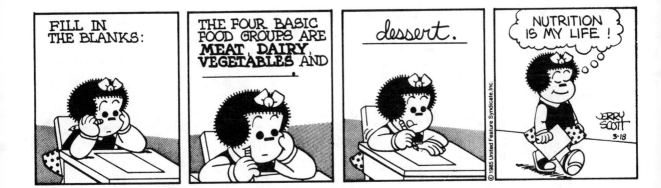

There are many good reasons to eat a healthy diet when you are trying to maintain weight. The first is that the right foods can make you feel better and give you more energy for life's activities. If you are eating less than you want, you may feel deprived and tired. When you restrict your calories, it is important to make good use of everything you eat.

Another reason to eat a balanced diet comes from a recent scientific discovery. The prevailing wisdom for many years was that a calorie is a calorie, no matter what food it comes from. People thought that eating 100 calories in lettuce was the same as 100 calories from pork chops. We now know that the body uses more energy (20-25% more) to metabolize carbohydrate than to metabolize the same number of calories of fat. Therefore, not only will eating a diet high in complex carbohydrates be more healthy than eating lots of fat, your body will burn more calories in the metabolic process.

The Concept of Caloric Density

Some foods are high in calories given their nutritional value. Soft drinks are an example. A can of Coke or Pepsi has about 140 calories, but there is no nutrition. If a person trying to keep to 1,200 calories per day drank 8 cans of soda, the day's calories would be shot and there would be no nutrients other than simple sugars.

A person who is restricting calories must be certain to make good use of the available calories. You have to cram all the nutrition you can into the calories you eat so that you get the proper mix of nutrients before exceeding the day's calorie level.

Here are several examples of high and low nutrient density. Fresh cherries will have greater nutrient density and lower caloric density than will cherry pie, because the pie has sugar and fat added to the cherries. Regular milk has greater nutrient density and lower caloric density than does chocolate milk, because the regular milk has the same nutrition with fewer calories. Popcorn with no butter is less dense with calories than buttered popcorn, which adds only fat.

cathy®   **by Cathy Guisewite**

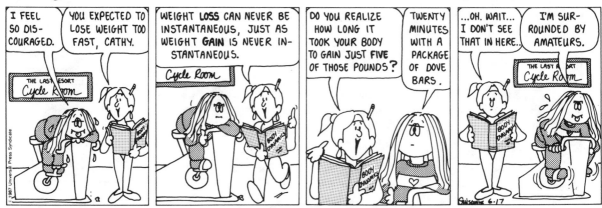

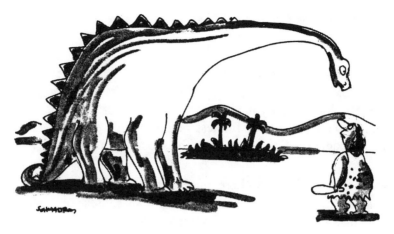

"How many calories are you?"

In general, eating a variety of healthy foods will insure that you have a nutritious diet. By following a few simple rules you can go a long way to having a healthier diet. An example of two such rules would be to eat less junk food and to eat more fruits and vegetables. It is important to be aware of the caloric density of foods, and to remember that every time you eat, you have an opportunity for good nutrition.

Making Every Calorie Count

When you are working to maintain weight loss, it is important to make certain that your calories bring good nutrition, and that you enjoy everything you eat. Going to a fast food place for the Ultra Monster Triple Bacon Cheeseburger might blow 2/3 of your day's calories. Sure -- it may taste good, but was it worth it? Does it justify having to eat almost nothing the rest of the day? Eating 14 of your Aunt Bertha's Chocolate Bomber Bon-Bons might feel good for the moment, but good enough?

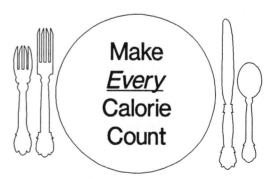

Here is where quantity control is the key. You need not deny yourself any food. However, eating large quantities at one time can be a waste of calories. Take Aunt Bertha's bon-bons for example. Would they bring you pleasure? Yes. Do they have much nutrition. No. Should you never have a single one? Probably not.

The issue, then, is how many bon-bons to eat. If we could attach a pleasure meter to your brain, we bet it would show an interesting picture. The first bon-bon would taste great -- the second one probably less so. As you get to bon-bon number 10, there would be little pleasure left, and the guilt and uncomfortable fullness would set in. Let's ask then, how many bon-bons were worth it? Probably the first, and maybe the second, but the rest? No way!

Laboratory studies show that there may be a biological basis for this. Food actually tastes less good as your biological state changes. As your body senses you have had enough, it helps control intake by making the food less pleasurable. Most people eat rapidly early in a meal and then slow down as the meal continues, perhaps because the food loses some of its appeal.

One trick to controlling weight is to make all your calories count. Don't eat beyond the point where you derive maximum pleasure (and sensible nutrition). How many potato chips are worth it? Can a few bites of ice cream or another dessert satisfy you as much as 30 bites? Each time you eat, think about the quality of the food, and about how much you need to feel good. Make the calories count.

Your Nutrition Savvy

Different people need different amounts of help with nutrition. Some are savvy and need little more than a refresher course. Others must start at scratch. Most fall in-between. In this chapter, we will help you determine where you stand with your nutrition knowledge, where to go for more help, and how to make food preparation interesting.

Take the Nutrition Quiz at the end of this Chapter. Answer all the questions before going over the answers that follow. After you take the Quiz, see how many correct responses you had.

The Quiz contains 19 questions. If you got 17 or more correct, you know your stuff. If you had fewer right than 17, some form of nutrition input would be helpful. The guidelines which follow describe where this input might be obtained. If you had many incorrect responses, don't worry. This is what happens to most people, and we designed the questions to be challenging.

Please bear in mind that this test cannot be used to assess your overall competence in nutrition. We chose questions that are relevant to health and weight control so that you could obtain a **general** idea of your knowledge.

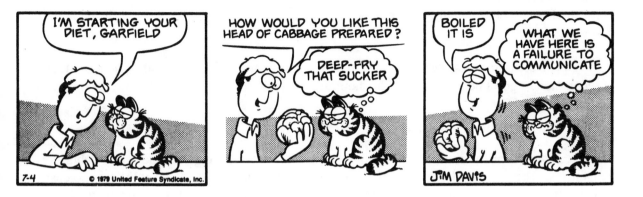

Keeping Sharp on Nutrition

At first glance, this would seem easy. Every bookstore has books on nutrition. The problem is that some of the books are wrong and may even be dangerous. What is a consumer to do?

First, you can be skeptical of books, programs, or people who promise miracle or breakthrough discoveries. Believe us, when such discoveries are made, you'll hear about them. Books that promise prolonged life, no risk for cancer, or remedies for other ailments should be viewed with great skepticism. Books that say that combining certain foods, eating foods in a certain order, eating some days and not others, or otherwise fiddling with what you know to be sound advice should be avoided.

Second, you can look to certain professionals or certain written materials for guidance. The suggestions that follow may be helpful in this regard. Because there are excellent resources available, we will help you identify the best approach for you from among the different approaches, rather than present a specific eating plan here. This way, you can identify the plan that will work best for you.

Seeing a Professional

For nutrition advice, a registered dietitian is usually the best person to see. This will be a person with an R.D. after her or his name. There are occasional people in other disciplines like medicine who know nutrition, but registered dietitians are trained to provide the type of advice you may need. They are expert at doing a nutritional assessment and can show you what nutrients you are getting in the foods you eat. They can also prescribe a healthy diet, usually with meal plans, recipes, and so forth.

You can contact a registered dietitian by looking in the Yellow Pages of the telephone book under "Dietitian," by asking your family physician, by calling the nearest hospital and asking for the Dietary Department, or by contacting the American Dietetic Association (listed in the next section).

The dietitian you see can provide intensive analysis and advice, or might do no more than recommend a good book. You and the dietitian can decide on the degree of input necessary.

Send For Available Materials

A wealth of information on healthy eating is available from government and voluntary agencies. These groups have booklets, brochures, and pamphlets available at little or no cost. The advice you will get from these materials will be sound, healthy, and straightforward. Here are some suggestions:

1)   **The American Heart Association**. Most cities have chapters of the American Heart Association (AHA). You can call or stop by the offices, explain that you are on a weight maintenance plan and would like materials on healthy eating. In addition, the AHA, which has its national headquarters in Dallas, has a toll free number to call to request information. This number is 1-800-242-2666. A diet that is "heart healthy" will be ideal for weight maintenance.

2)   **The American Cancer Society**. The American Cancer Society (ACS) also has branches around the country, so check the telephone directory and call to see how you might obtain information. In addition, the national headquarters of the ACS has a toll-free number to call for information. It is 1-800-628-3790. An "anti-cancer" diet will be quite similar to a heart healthy diet, so information from either of the agencies shown here will be valuable.

3)   **The National Heart, Lung, and Blood Institute**. This is one of the branches of the National Institutes of Health in Bethesda, Maryland. This government agency is the primary sponsor of research programs on heart disease. The Institute has materials available on diet and healthy eating. Information on these can be obtained by calling 301-951-3260.

4)   **The National Cancer Institute**. Also a branch of the National Institutes of Health in Bethesda, Maryland, this is the main government agency concerned with the control of cancer. Because dietary factors have been implicated in cancer, the NCI has developed materials on diet and healthy eating. Information can be obtained by calling the Cancer Information Service toll free at 1-800-422-6237.

5)   **The American Dietetic Association**. The ADA is the nation's largest group of food and nutrition professionals, with more than 59,000 members, most of whom are registered dietitians. The ADA has information available on nutrition and on how to locate a dietitian for professional advice. The ADA is at 216 West Jackson Blvd., Chicago, IL 60606-6995 (telephone is 312-899-0040). Among their materials, the ADA has a pamphlet published in 1990 called "10 Tips to Healthy Eating."

Getting A Good Book

There are a number of good books available on eating in a healthy fashion. As we mentioned before, it is not always easy to separate the good from the bad when you stroll through the bookstore, so here are some recommendations. Some might be available when you shop, but all can be ordered. Just ask at the counter.

a)   Brody J. *Jane Brody's Good Food Book.* New York: Bantam Books, 1987.

b)   DeBakey ME, Gotto AM, Scott LW, Foreyt JP. *The Living Heart Diet.* New York: Simon & Schuster, 1984.

c)   Goor R, Goor N. *Eater's Choice: A Food Lover's Guide to Lower Cholesterol.* Boston: Houghton-Mifflin, 1987.

d)   Saltman P, Gurin J, Mothner I. *The California Nutrition Book.* Boston: Little Brown, 1987.

Making It Interesting

Just knowing the right foods to eat does not guarantee that the eating will be interesting. It is easy to fall into the trap of having good food made in a boring way. It is quite possible to prepare food in interesting, varied, and nutritious ways. The books that follow contain many mouth-watering recipes. If you try them, you may find your new diet more interesting than the old.

a)   American Heart Association. *American Heart Association Cookbook (4th ed.).* New York: McKay, 1984.

b)   American Heart Association. *American Heart Association Low-Fat, Low-Cholesterol Cookbook.* New York: Times Books, 1989.

c)   Better Homes and Gardens. *Better Homes and Gardens Diet Recipes.* Des Moines, Iowa: Meredith, 1986.

d)   *Betty Crocker's Eat and Lose Weight.* New York: Prentice-Hall, 1990.

e)   Brody J. *Jane Brody's Good Food Book.* New York: Bantam Books, 1987.

f)   *Cooking Light Cookbook.* Birmingham, AL: Oxmoor House, 1989.

g)   DeBakey, ME, Gotto AM, Scott LW, Foreyt JP. *The Living Heart Diet.* New York: Simon & Schuster, 1984.

h)   Kafka, B. *Microwave Gourmet Lifestyle Cookbook.* New York: Morrow, 1989.

i)   Madison D, Brown EE. *The Greens Cookbook: Extraordinary Vegetarian Cuisine from The Celebrated Restaurant.* New York: Bantam Books, 1987.

j)   Rodale Publishers. *Rodale's Garden Fresh Cooking.* Emmaus, PA : Rodale Press, 1987.

k)   Weight Watchers. *Weight Watchers Quick and Easy Menu Cookbook.* New York: New American Library, 1987.

l)   Weight Watchers. *Weight Watchers Meals in Minutes Cookbook.* New York: New American Library, 1989.

The Best System For Good Nutrition

There are several good systems for eating nutritiously. One system is a calorie counting plan where you learn to count calories and choose a specified number of servings from the basic food groups.

The second system, which is also widely used, is the exchange plan developed by the American Dietetic Association and the American Diabetes Association. In this plan, you select a certain number of exchanges from basic food groups. You can exchange foods within a food group (e.g., milk may be substituted for yogurt), but the object is to have the specified number of exchanges in each group.

The two approaches are both good ones. You will find detailed information on both in the materials mentioned earlier in this chapter. We recommend you contact the organizations we listed and check out the nutrition books and cookbooks we cited. These will help you keep weight off and to eat well in the process.

As a helpful starting point, we would like to offer some guidelines developed jointly by the American Dietetic Association and the International Food Information Council. These "10 Tips to Healthy Eating" provide a healthy, balanced approach that will help you stay healthy and control your weight.

10
Tips To Healthy Eating

1. Eat a variety of nutrient-rich foods.

2. Enjoy plenty of whole grains, fruits, and vegetables.

3. Maintain a healthy body weight.

4. Eat moderate portions.

5. Eat regular meals.

6. Reduce, don't eliminate, certain foods.

7. Balance your food choices over time.

8. Know your diet pitfalls.

9. Make changes gradually.

10. Remember, foods are not good or bad.

Source: The American Dietetic Association
and the International Food Information Council

Nutrition Quiz

		True	False
1.	The calorie is the measure of the amount of fat in food.	____	____
2.	Eating an extra 10 calories per day will add one pound of weight over a year.	____	____
3.	The four food groups are Dairy Products, Fruits and Vegetables, Breads and Cereals, and Meats and Proteins.	____	____
4.	If you eat an equal number of servings from the four food groups, you will have a balanced diet.	____	____
5.	Meat, fish, eggs, poultry, and milk are good sources of protein.	____	____
6.	One ounce of fat contains twice the calories of one ounce of sugar.	____	____
7.	Fat soluble vitamins give you energy, but water soluble vitamins do not.	____	____
8.	Vitamin B_{12} is the only vitamin for which mega-doses are recommended.	____	____
9.	Alcohol is dangerous for dieters because it contains many calories and weakens dietary restraint.	____	____
10.	Vitamin E is associated with virility and may help in the remedy of alcoholism.	____	____
11.	Fruits, vegetables, and cereals tend to be high in fiber.	____	____
12.	For controlling your blood cholesterol, it is important to limit intake of saturated fat.	____	____
13.	The average person consumes more than twice the safe and adequate intake of salt each day.	____	____
14.	Foods obtained from plants have no cholesterol, whereas those from animals do.	____	____
15.	Whole grain products mainly provide simple carbohydrates.	____	____
16.	To gain one pound, you have to eat 3,500 calories more than you burn.	____	____
17.	Vegetable fats are usually unsaturated fats.	____	____
18.	Dietary fiber is a form of protein.	____	____
19.	Polyunsaturated fat lowers cholesterol levels in the blood.	____	____

Answers To Nutrition Quiz

1. *False*   The calorie is a measure of the energy your body gets from food. Fat supplies some of these calories in some foods, but so do carbohydrate and protein.

2. *True*   As few as 10 calories make a difference when added over a period like a year.

3. *True*   These are the four food groups. In order to have a balanced diet, a variety of foods should be eaten from these groups.

4. *False*   Different numbers of servings are recommended for the four groups.

5. *True*   These are good sources of protein, which is an essential nutrient for the body.

6. *True*   Fat has twice the calories as carbohydrates or protein. Decreasing the fat in your diet can really help with weight loss.

7. *False*   Vitamins do not produce energy themselves, but aid in the breakdown of other nutrients into energy the body can use.

8. *False*   There is no advantage to taking mega-doses of any vitamin. Sticking with the Recommended Daily Allowance (RDA) is the best policy. This can usually be done by eating a balanced diet, and at most, can be accomplished with a multiple vitamin.

9. *True*   Alcohol releases inhibitions and weakens dietary restraint. It contains little nutrition and many calories.

10. *False*   Unless you are vitamin deficient or have special dietary needs, you probably need no vitamin supplements. A balanced diet usually provides adequate vitamins.

11. *True*   These foods are naturally high in fiber and are good additions to your diet if you wish to increase fiber intake.

12. *True*   Saturated fat can raise your cholesterol level, so it is important to control the intake of foods high in cholesterol *and* foods high in saturated fat.

13. *True*   Most experts recommend reductions in salt intake. Excess sodium comes from salt in foods naturally and from the salt we add to food.

14. *True*   This is why foods from plant sources (like margarine) are better choices than similar foods from animal sources (like butter).

15. *False*   Whole grain products are a good source of complex carbohydrates, which are useful for dieting.

16. *True*   The general rule of thumb is that one pound of fat stores about 3,500 calories.

Answers To Nutrition Quiz (continued)

17. *True*   Unsaturated fats are better than saturated fats, so like your mother told you, "Eat your vegetables."

18. *False*   Fiber is a source of carbohydrate.

19. *True*   It is advisable to consume more unsaturated fat than saturated fat. Saturated fat can increase blood cholesterol levels.

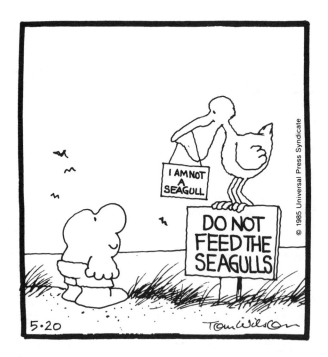

CHAPTER NINE

The Power of Positive Thinking

When a drug company wants to test a new medication, it often uses a double blind procedure. That is, half the test group is given the medicine, while the other half is given a placebo, an inactive pill containing only sugar or some other harmless substance. Neither the researcher nor the individuals in the test program know which group is getting the real drug and which is getting the placebo until the results are tallied. The odd thing is that the results are often as good or better in the group receiving the placebo as in the group receiving the medicine. This sometimes happens because the drugs don't work, but more often because amazing things occur when people **believe** things will change.

Mind Over Matter

There is now a great deal of research indicating that the mind has a mysterious power over the body. In one study, researchers found that people felt much better after they had been to a clinic to see their doctor. Then the scientists tested people who were still in the waiting room and they felt better too. Finally they tested people who hadn't come to the clinic, but had made an appointment. They felt better already. Clearly your thoughts can operate in your service. But they can also operate in your disservice.

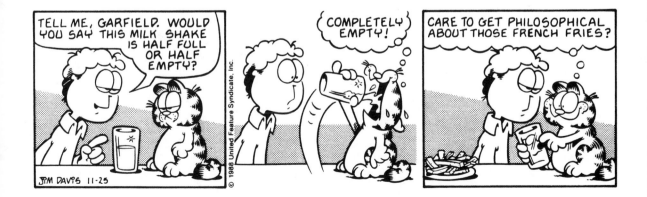

Psychologists believe that your thought patterns control your behavior. The exciting thing is that you can change many of your thoughts by changing your self-statements. Self-statements are the things you say to yourself about yourself.

At first, it is not easy to change your self-statements, but it gets easier with practice. By becoming aware of what you are thinking and feeling, you can identify how your thoughts turn you on to eating. You will be following essentially the same process you used to identify your external eating triggers. But this time you won't have to cope with outside events or people you can't change, because the same thoughts that now may be working against you can be developed to work for you.

Your Mental Tape

Think of your mind as a recording tape that plays back a phrase. If making negative self-statements is one of your problems, you can learn to erase that tape and record new positive statements.

Suppose, for instance, you've eaten something inconsistent with your plan. The mental tape recorder says disapprovingly, "You stupid jerk, you've blown it again. No wonder you're so disgustingly fat." This negative self-statement will inevitably lead you to overeat more. Erase that tape and record a new message. "O.K. I took in 400 extra calories. To come out even, I'll eat 250 fewer calories tomorrow and walk a little more for the next week."

The first tape is what we call a maladaptive cognition. By calling yourself bad, you actually give yourself permission to **be** bad. Add that to the guilt you feel, and you've got a situation ripe for overeating. The new recording is an adaptive cognition. It accepts responsibility for the problem but then includes a realistic strategy to compensate for it.

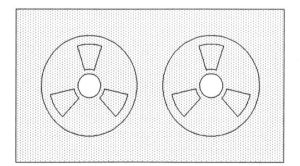

Erasing Your Mental Tape

Re-Recording Your Tape

Listen to your own tape. Whenever you put yourself down, say something more helpful. Helpful thoughts include a goal, and an action to achieve your goal.

Here is a list of some bad thoughts, and some good thoughts that could be used instead. Remember that good thoughts are those that accept responsibility for the action but then include a realistic strategy to compensate for it.

Bad Thoughts	Good Thoughts
1.	_If I overeat, I say to myself:_
"Oh no, I've blown it"	"I was too hungry. Next time I must eat lunch if I know dinner will be so late."
2.	_If I don't like how I look, I say to myself:_
"You fat pig, what's wrong with you?	"I will not wear clothes with stripes running horizontally."
3.	_If I have had a fight with a friend, I say to myself:_
"You jerk, why can't you get along with anyone?"	"Next time I will discuss my bad feelings before I explode in anger."

Now you try one:

You come home after fighting traffic and almost having an accident. You devour a plate of cookies and then say to yourself: "You're hardly in the door and now you're eating cookies. You can't even deal with the simplest things."

_____

_____

_____

Example: "Traffic was insane today and I drove as well as I could. I know I eat without thinking when I'm tense, so instead of eating cookies, I'll go for a walk the next time I'm tense."

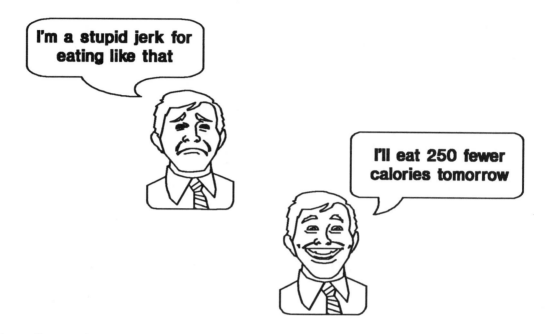

Auto-Suggestion

During the 1920's, a French psychotherapist named Emil Coue' became world famous as a proponent of auto-suggestion. Millions of Americans followed his teaching by repeating to themselves: "Every day, in every way, I am getting better and better." Like all fads it died out, but the doctor had a good point. Modern research confirms that, to a significant degree, you are what you tell yourself you are because your perceptions and interpretations strongly affect your behavior. That's why saying positive things about yourself is so important.

To be positive you have to eliminate critical judgments against yourself and your behavior, and replace them with a realistic plan for action. When you make positive self-statements you are less likely to make negative ones. It's easy to tell them apart. Negative self-statements are put-downs that blame but don't solve anything. Positive self-statements are goal-directed. They acknowledge responsibility and include a positive, realistic idea for what you can do next time.

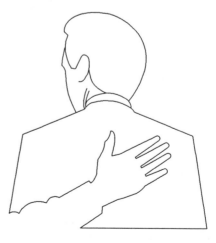

Patting Yourself On The Back

Using Positive Self-Statements in High-Risk Areas

When you think about your high-risk areas, you may feel that problems are inevitable. For instance, when you come home after a hard day, you might think it's inevitable that you scout around the kitchen for something to eat. But suppose you break the chain of events into its component parts. You may discover that you can change one of those parts quite easily, by changing how you think. For instance, if you leave the office tense after a hard day at work, and think about food all the way home, you will head straight for the refrigerator. You wolf down something and then you blame yourself. Your guilt then leads to more eating.

Positive Self-Statements Are

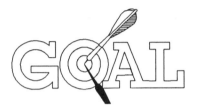

Goal Directed

Where did the problem start? Where can you break this chain? The tension you felt at the start is the best signal. If you use techniques to get rid of the tension, you can break the chain at its first link. But suppose you don't. Other parts of the sequence can be interrupted too. For instance, you can change your mental TV channel. Don't think about food on the way home after a high stress day. Shift your attention to pleasurable, non-food thoughts.

Another part of the chain, later on, involves guilt and self-blame. Here, replacing negative self-statements with positive ones is the key. Use the open refrigerator door as a red light. Do not wage a moral war with yourself, saying "What's wrong with me, I can't believe I am doing this." Instead, try more positive self-statements. "What is the texture I am craving"? or "If I still want a piece of pie in an hour I can have it," or "Maybe an apple will satisfy this need to eat."

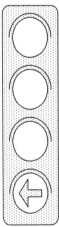

Pay Attention To Signals

With awareness, you can identify the elements, single out the ones you can control, and break the chain. The first step in high-risk situations is identifying and defining all the elements that went into making up the problem. We talk more about high-risk situations in Chapter 3.

Practice Breaking The Chain

Here are two case histories: Susan and Fran. In Susan's case, she was able to deal successfully with her problem situations in a variety of ways. Analyze the chain of events in her story, breaking it down into separate parts. Identify the strategies she used to cope with the stresses and temptations of the day.

SUSAN: CASE EPISODE

Susan wakes up in the morning, takes a shower, and brushes her teeth. She takes a couple of minutes while getting dressed to preplan what she will eat that day. She also tries to identify any foreseeable situations that may interfere with her plans. She remembers that she is going out to lunch with a friend who always chooses a restaurant that doesn't serve the kind of food that Susan wants to eat. She rehearses how she will respond to her friend's suggestion that they go to the usual restaurant. She dresses, eats breakfast, and leaves for work.

At the office, Susan has a terrible morning. She can't believe how unfair everyone is being. When the coffee break rolls around, she knows there are doughnuts in the next room. She can't stop herself from going to look at them, but she pictures them swimming in dirty globs of grease. She feels disgusted and decides to take a walk instead of eating. She thinks about how much more she enjoyed the walk than she would have enjoyed a doughnut.

Lunchtime comes. Susan tells her friend that she would like to go to a restaurant where they can both find food that they want, and her friend agrees.

Back at the office after lunch, Susan finds out that she will have to work quite late. A friend is expecting to go shopping with her at 7:00, so she calls to reschedule their shopping for the next day. This way Susan will have time to exercise at the gym.

Now read Fran's case history. Fran was not successful at dealing with her problem situations. Analyze the events in her day, breaking them down into separate parts. For Fran, recommend thought and self-statement strategies she might have used to cope with her day's events.

FRAN: CASE EPISODE

Fran's friends plan a weekend in New York. She's eager to join them although she worries about how she will control the usual food orgies involved in their New York visits. Too rushed for breakfast, they grab coffee and doughnuts at the train station. Fran refuses but she's starving by the time she gets to New York. It still is two hours until lunch time and her friends don't want to waste time eating so they spend the rest of the morning rushing frantically around the stores. Fran is exhausted as well as famished. Finally, they agree to eat lunch. They suggest pizza. Fran agrees reluctantly, promising herself that she will have only one piece of the pizza.

After a long wait for the pizza to be served, Fran is beside herself. She eats her slice of pizza very quickly and feels that she is still hungry after only one piece. Everyone else is continuing to eat. She decides to have one more piece of pizza, resolving to be very good later on tonight. She asks for the platter to be passed to her, and quickly eats a second piece of the pie. The aroma from the pizza platter that is now in front of her is too much to resist, so she has another piece, and still another. After her fourth piece of pizza, Fran is furious at herself. The friends leave the pizza parlor.

As they walk down the street, they see a pastry shop and decide to go in for coffee. The waiter invites them to browse at the pastry counter before ordering. Fran tells herself that she wants to enjoy this day and that it will be the last time she eats fattening food this month. She orders a pastry with her coffee.

The friends spend the afternoon at a movie. They pass the tub (the extra large size) of buttered popcorn back and forth and Fran feels angry at them for tempting her. She resists but her fury mounts and she can barely concentrate on the show. "Why don't they care more about me"? she complains inwardly. "If they did, they'd understand how I'm feeling."

Here are some ideas, to go along with your own, of what Fran might have done:

Fran might have chosen something low in calories to buy at the train station. She could even have eaten a piece of the doughnut if that was her only choice. By going hungry, she was setting herself up for problems later in the day.

Fran should have suggested an alternative to pizza. If her friends were unwilling, she might have been satisfied with less pizza if she had eaten breakfast.

Telling yourself "this is the last time for fattening food this month" is a sure set-up for failure. Fran wanted the pastry because she felt bad for eating the pizza. If she had eaten too much pizza, she needed to tell herself at the pastry shop that the pizza was high in calories, but OK as long as she didn't go overboard for the rest of the day. Then she might only have ordered coffee.

Finally at the movies, Fran was making many negative self-statements. Positive self-statements would be a great help to her here. For example, she might say "I will get a diet soft-drink and pass up the popcorn. I'm certainly not hungry. If my friends want to ruin their dinner, that's their problem, but I will not."

Attributions

Attributions are the explanations that you give yourself, regarding your own behavior. Often when things happen we ask ourselves, "Why did I do it,?" or "Why did that happen?" The explanations that we give ourselves have a profound effect on our next actions.

Changing Explanations

For successful maintenance you need to change attributions about your weight and body, about food and potential high-risk situations, and about yourself in general. Rather than blaming yourself for failures, look for explanations for your failures in the situations you are facing.

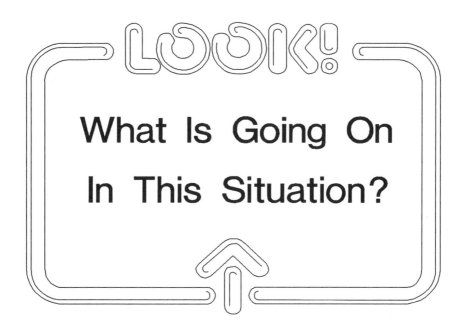

We have already seen how this works in helping you to change negative self-statements into positive self-statements. All of the "good" thoughts we listed dealt with things in the situation that could be changed or aspects of your behavior that could be modified. The "bad" thoughts focused on stable characteristics that were hard to change and were derogatory.

You are not trying to be a Pollyanna. You are simply learning how to think more helpfully by finding explanations for your behaviors that provide opportunities for change.

Your Mental Television Screen

Perhaps there are mental images that trigger strong hunger for you. Passing a Baskin Robbins or Howard Johnson's, or merely hearing their name, may cause an image to appear on your mental television screen in full glorious color. It's a giant chocolate sundae topped with whipped cream and a cherry.

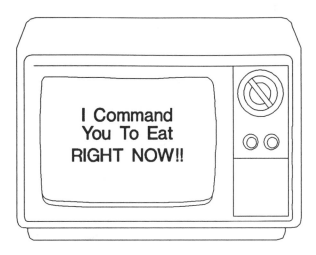

Changing the Channel

Here are three examples of ways to change your mental images: Rather than let the food image stimulate your desire to eat, you can train your brain to change the image to something unrelated to food. For example, all at once the mound of ice cream could change into a beautiful mountain against a blue sky. What looked like whipped cream on top is really snow and that red cherry at the peak is the setting sun just about to sink below the mountain top. Instead of thinking about eating, you're on a rewarding mental vacation trip.

Perhaps your Aunt Mary phones and her voice evokes memories. Suddenly you picture her offering a plate of whipped potatoes swimming in her famous pot roast gravy. Instead try to think of the plate as a sculpture that doesn't look at all edible.

You're reading a magazine article. The writer describes a dessert he had in a restaurant in France. Suddenly it appears in graphic detail on your mental television screen -- a multi-layered chocolate torte, frosted with little sprinkles of chocolate. But wait. Didn't one of those sprinkles move? Yes, they are all moving. They're ants. Disgusting!

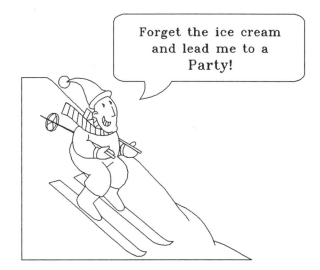

Use your ability to conjure up images to your advantage, rather than to your disadvantage. There are at least three ways to avoid visual "turn-ons".

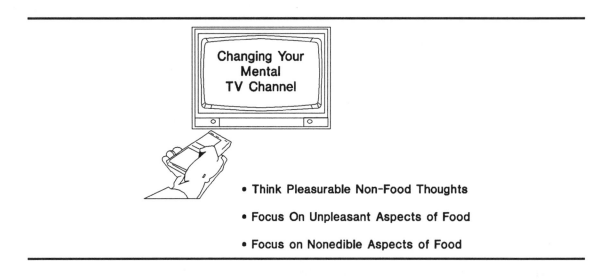

- Think Pleasurable Non-Food Thoughts

- Focus On Unpleasant Aspects of Food

- Focus on Nonedible Aspects of Food

Summary

We've reviewed many ways that your thoughts can help or hinder your maintenance efforts. While there are no inflexible prescriptions, in general the following "don'ts and do's" should work for you.

Don'ts

☐   **Avoid setting unreasonable goals**
☐   **Avoid negative self-statements**
☐   **Avoid words like "always" and "never"**
☐   **Don't call yourself "stupid" or "bad"**

Do's

☐   **Make positive self-statements that include concrete plans for action**
☐   **Think about progress, not shortcomings**
☐   **Look for problems in situations, not only in yourself**
☐   **Use imagery techniques to change your mental channels**

CHAPTER TEN

Social Bonds and Your Weight: Can Others Help?

Social Factors and Health

First a point, then an explanation.

You would be amazed at the role social factors play in our emotions and our health. Have you heard stories of an elderly person dying and then their spouse dying shortly after? Did you know that married men live longer than single men, and that social disruption such as divorce, moving, or death of a loved one increases the chance of illness?

Not only can social factors influence **whether** a person gets ill, but whether and how quickly they **recover** once they are ill. Having a good social network can help in recovery from chronic diseases such as cancer and heart disease.

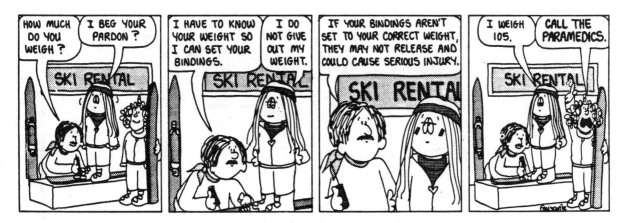

Researchers at the University of California at Berkeley showed how important these factors are in a study in Northern California. They collected information on approximately 7,000 individuals to see which lifestyle factors related to risk of serious disease. These researchers developed an index of social support for each person based on four factors: marriage, contact with close friends and neighbors, church affiliation, and formal and informal group associations. People with higher scores on this index lived longer than people with less supportive social networks.

Why It Works

Now that we agree that social support is important, why does it work? There are several theories about this, each of them interesting.

The first possibility is that social support improves health directly. Because of the steadying influence it has, positive relationships with others might keep the body more relaxed, less weakened by worry and other negative feelings, and better prepared to fight off disease, perhaps through a better functioning immune system.

The second possibility is that social support buffers a person against difficult life events and the accompanying stress. If this is true, support doesn't make you healthier *per se*, but it protects you against the negative health effects of stressful life events. Everybody encounters such events, but some people come unglued while others recover quickly. Social support might be one factor that softens the blow.

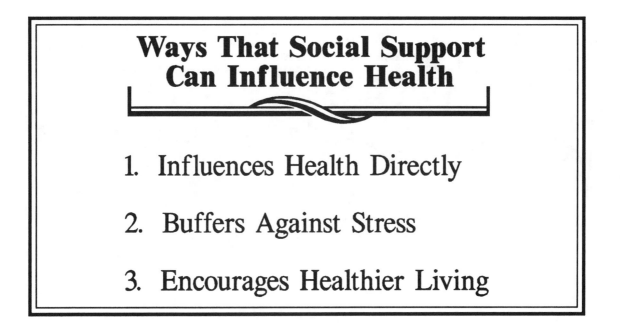

Ways That Social Support Can Influence Health

1. Influences Health Directly

2. Buffers Against Stress

3. Encourages Healthier Living

Social Support

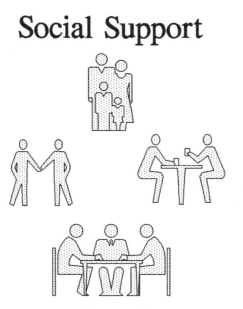

The third possibility is that social support provides an incentive to adopt a healthier lifestyle. A man who has a wife and children, for example, might have a special incentive to not smoke and to eat a healthy diet. A woman who has support from others might feel better about herself and work to take extra care of her body.

Science cannot yet tell us which of these explanations or combinations of explanations best explains why social support and good health go together. Our intuition and clinical judgement tell us that all are correct, at least to some extent. This is good news for someone trying to control their weight, because learning to elicit support from others around you may help you maintain your weight. Remember one thing. Knowing that support can help is one thing. The challenge is to get it to work for you, not against you.

Who Needs Support?

From the above discussion, you would expect the answer to this question to be "everybody." Not so with weight control. Some people take to support like a bee to honey, but others don't respond and may even find it troubling to have others involved in their program. Here is the place to see which applies to you.

Solo Vs. Social Weight Control

In our experience, people differ in how they view support from others. Some are sociable about their eating and weight, while others want these to be private. We call these two types **solo** and **social** maintainers.

Social maintainers want others involved in what they do. They tell other people they are watching their weight and are able to talk about their successes and setbacks. They may like to be complimented and may post a graph of their weight change in a visible location. They might prefer a group program to an individual program and might prefer to exercise with others rather than exercise alone.

Solo maintainers are much different. They do not want others involved with their weight maintenance program. They prefer to exercise alone and don't necessarily want others talking to them about their program. They may function well in a group, but be able to take or leave the social aspects.

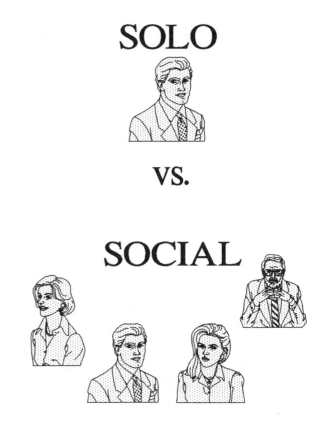

By now, you may have already decided which of these two categories best fits you. Many people relate instantly to one of these descriptions. Even if this is true of you, fill out the Social vs. Solo Inventory given on the following page. This will help you decide which style is the "real you."

After you complete the quiz, see how many true and false answers you had. The more true answers you selected, the more you are a social maintainer. If many of your answers were false, the solo category might fit better.

Which Is Best?

Now that you know whether you are more of a social or solo maintainer, it is important to understand that neither is best -- they are just different. Social maintainers can have great success with this program, and so can solo maintainers. If you are the solo type, fine. You can maintain your weight loss and there is no need to force the issue of social support. If you are a social maintainer, fine. You can do well also, but you have an additional resource within your reach. We will teach you how to reach out and grab it.

Social Vs. Solo Inventory

		Ture	False
1.	I talk to other people about my weight.	_____	_____
2.	Given a choice, I would rather exercise with others than alone.	_____	_____
3.	I would rather have people compliment me on my weight change than leave me alone.	_____	_____
4.	I feel I could talk to a close friend about my weight and my eating.	_____	_____
5.	I can accept positive comments from others.	_____	_____
6.	In a weight loss program, I would do just fine in a group.	_____	_____
7.	I like others to notice when I am doing well with my weight.	_____	_____
8.	I consider myself more of a sociable person than a loner.	_____	_____
9.	I like to be around other people.	_____	_____
10.	With regard to weight maintenance, I would like to have others support me.	_____	_____

Here is why we believe these two types are different, but equal. One of us (KDB) did several of the first studies on social support and weight loss. In these studies, some dieters attended meetings alone while others involved their spouses. The theory was that those who had their spouses involved would do better because of the additional support. Funny thing was, the studies yielded inconsistent results. Some found a big advantage for the spouse groups, but others did not. In the studies showing an advantage for spouse groups, the additional weight loss was not evident during the initial program, but was evident during **maintenance**.

After a number of studies were done, it became more clear why the results were inconsistent. For social individuals, having a spouse involved is a positive, supportive experience. For solo people, this is intrusive and creates conflict. Consequently, having others involved works fine for some, but not for others. It is important for you to decide whether the social or solo approach is best for you.

Some programs ignore social support while others push it for everyone. An example of the later philosophy are programs that require all participants to team up with another person in a buddy system. This works fine for swimmers at summer camp, but not always for people trying to control their weight. Forcing this on a solo maintainer is like forcing a square peg into a round hole.

The information that follows is aimed at people who feel they may benefit from support from others. These guidelines will help show you when support is needed and how to get it.

As a special note, even if you believe you are a solo maintainer, read on. There may come a time when you feel that others can help, or there might be isolated circumstances when input from another person might be beneficial. Knowing what to do when the right conditions arise will permit you to respond effectively.

When Do You Need Support?

We want to point out again that support is a resource that can be used in different ways by different people. One way is to have support around you all the time. This might be accomplished by working on maintenance with a partner, or having a spouse or good friend very involved in your program. The support is available when you do well and when you have trouble. The supporting people know how you are doing and can be helpful on a regular basis.

Support can also be used for crisis intervention. Some people have support available and even lined up, but call on it only in a crisis. Such a person might call on others for support when they have had an eating binge, when they feel that control is slipping, when they miss program meetings, or when they have a strong urge to eat.

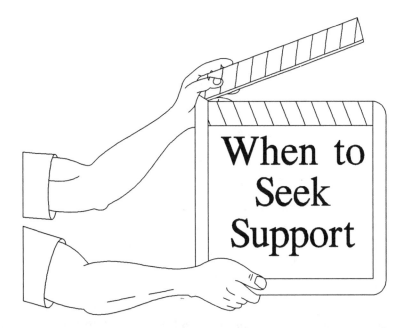

In applying the information that follows, think about how you would like support to best help you. Some people begin by enlisting support more continuously but then make the transition to support on an "as needed" basis. This makes sense because once a person gets to know their triggers for eating, and is sensitive to high-risk situations, support might only be required sporadically. Sometimes just knowing it's there makes a difference.

Avoiding Social Situations

Some individuals avoid social situations because they are embarrassed and ashamed about their weight. If you still have weight to lose, you may feel the same. The case of Bonnie is a classic example.

Bonnie was in one of our groups and was losing, but not as quickly as she wanted. As she began to feel more comfortable with the group, she explained some of the sad ways her weight had influenced her life. Her husband, who was thin, was embarrassed to be seen with her. Even though he had worked at his job for more than 12 years, Bonnie had been to no social gatherings of office people and had met none of his coworkers. When her husband went to these gatherings, he made excuses that Bonnie was sick, visiting relatives, or working.

We might expect Bonnie to be resentful about this, and she was. However, she was also ashamed herself, and in one way, it was easier for her to stay home and not worry about facing people. She and her husband had an unspoken pact where they both agreed that she should be punished for being heavy.

Avoiding Social Situations

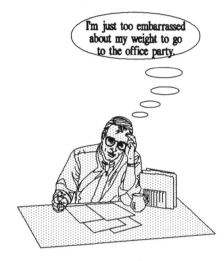

It is a mistake to put your social life on hold because you weigh more than you'd like. Here are the reasons. First, **there is much more to life than weight**. We are hoping this book will help you put weight into perspective. We realize that it may be important to you, but not so important that thinking about it and working on it overwhelms the rest of your life. Second, if you never quite lose all the weight you intend to lose, will you avoid social situations forever?

There are many heavy people who have lost some, but not all of the weight they would like. They have accepted their weight and shape and lead fulfilling, satisfying lives. They are good at their jobs, are good parents, and have satisfying relationships with family and friends. Even something that you might believe would be hampered by excess weight, like a good sex life, can be terrific if people accept their bodies and have a loving partner.

The moral to this story is simple. Avoiding social situations will make a person resentful. They will resent themselves for being the way they are and will resent others who encourage this to happen. It is possible to feel good about yourself at any weight. Avoiding social situations will make you feel worse about your weight. Even more important, it will keep you away from the very people who might help you with your efforts at weight control. Read on to learn more.

Being In Groups

Groups provide an excellent source of social support for some people. Other people in a group can provide much in the way of help and support. On the help side, other people may have been through the same things you face, and may have useful solutions. They can be the source of good ideas on many aspects of diet and nutrition. You would be surprised at the clever ideas your fellow group members can have.

On the support side, groups can be invaluable because of the caring, understanding, and encouragement that members give each other. Being around people with a similar situation shows that you are not the only one in the world with a certain problem. Knowing that others are in the same boat allows you to help them and them to help you.

Evidence for the power of groups is shown by the self-help movement. People have organized self-help groups for almost everything. There are groups for those who have lost loved ones, have certain diseases, have problems with drugs, alcohol, and gambling and even for those raised in families with some of these problems. These groups provide great help to many people, including some who do not fancy themselves as the type for groups.

For the person wanting to lose or maintain weight, there are many groups available. This is good news because the options are extensive and there is a good chance that you can find something to suit you.

Many hospitals and clinics have group weight loss programs. These are usually run by a health professional such as a dietitian, nurse, psychologist, physician, or exercise specialist. These groups can provide support as well as useful information.

Many of the commercial weight loss programs have groups. Weight Watchers is the classic example. The Weight Watchers meetings have a leader and members of a group. In some cases the groups are large and are more like a class or lecture, but in other cases, the groups are small enough to permit interaction among the members.

Overeaters Anonymous (OA) and Take Off Pounds Sensibly (TOPS) are examples of self-help groups. The groups are usually small and people are free to speak as they wish. In OA, each member can have a sponsor, who is another person in the group they can call at any time for support and guidance. Leaders in commercial, and self-help groups are typically not professionals, but volunteers or paid staff who may have lost weight on the program themselves.

How do you know if you are a group person? One way is to try different groups and see how you respond. If you have been in programs in the past, think back on your experience. Did you feel supported having others in the group working on similar problems?

The best way to know if a group is for you is to decide what it is you need to control your weight and if this can be obtained from a group. Some individuals need to be accountable and feel they must be weighed by someone on a regular basis. Some people like the ideas and information that come from a group. Others like the social climate of being around other people. For yet others, it is the supportive environment and words of encouragement that make the group so important. Decide if these things are important for you. There are some dieters who may not like groups particularly, but still find that they are important in their weight control efforts.

If a group does have the potential to help you, it is time to find the right group for **you**. The best way to do this is to be a smart consumer. Visit the nearby programs and see if you can sit in on a group, or at least talk to the people who run the program. Find the right mix of people, the right size group, and the right focus for the group. For example, some focus on compulsive eating (like OA), others focus on specific foods or supplements offered by the program, and still others focus on education in behavior change, exercise, and nutrition.

One aspect of choosing the right group lies in the decision about how you should best use the group. One way is to join a group with a definite beginning and ending time, like a hospital program where you begin the program with a certain group of people and then stick with the same group for the duration of the program (usually three or four months). Another way is to wait until you really need the support and then join. A third way is to use a program for crisis intervention. Attending a Weight Watchers group is something you could hold in reserve until a crisis arises, then you could attend several meetings, stop going, and begin again when the need arises.

As a final note, group support can also be obtained in exercise programs. Joining a health club can provide a new series of contacts, and most clubs have group activities such as aerobics classes. These classes are also available in local churches, schools, YMCA's and so forth. If you have trouble exercising regularly on your own, this is an excellent way to provide a social incentive.

Weight Maintenance With a Partner

Weight partnerships are when two people or more decide to lose or maintain weight at the same time and to work together. These partnerships can be very powerful if the right chemistry exists between the people and if each knows what to do to support the other.

The first step is to decide whether a partnership would work for you. Have you tried anything like this in the past and how did it work? Can you see yourself talking with such a person frequently about your program? Knowing that a partner would be supporting you, would you be able to support the partner in return? Do you think a partner would provide a boost to your motivation during difficult times?

Maintenance Partnership

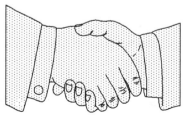

If you feel a partner may help, the next step is to find the right partner. This can be a spouse, coworker, neighbor, friend, relative, or even someone who lives some distance from you but is in close contact. The main issue is whether you feel comfortable with each other and have close and frequent contact.

Think for a moment of people who might be good partners for you. Think about how you two relate and whether the relationship is friendly and supportive enough to work together on something that will endure for weeks or even months. Then, fill out the Partnership Quiz which is provided on the next page.

The Partnership Quiz is taken from *The LEARN™ Program For Weight Control* (by Brownell). It was designed to help an individual decide whether a specific person would make a good diet partner. It can also be used to help find a good maintenance partner. Think of a person who might make a good partner, and then fill out the quiz. Below each question is a number. Add the numbers of the responses you checked, then use the following scoring guide:

If you scored between 30 and 34, you may have found the perfect partner. A score in this range indicates that you and your friend are comfortable with one another and can work together.

If you scored between 25 and 29, your friend is potentially a good partner, but there are a few areas of concern. Try asking the partner to take the quiz and predict how you answered the questions. This may help you make a decision.

If you scored between 17 and 24, there are potential areas of conflict, and a diet partnership could encounter stormy going. Think of another partner.

If you scored between 8 and 16, definitely look to someone else as a partner. A diet partnership in this case would be a high-risk undertaking.

The Partnership Quiz should help you identify an individual who might be a helpful maintenance partner. Remember that this approach is not for everyone, but it might work for you. If so, the next section gives some guidelines for making social support work for you.

Partnership Quiz

		True	False
1.	It is easy to talk to my partner about weight.	5	1
2.	My partner has always been thin and does not understand my weight problem.	1	3
3.	My partner offers me food when he or she knows I am on a diet.	1	5
4.	My partner never says critical things about my weight.	3	1
5.	My partner is always there when I need a friend.	4	1
6.	When I lose weight and look better, my partner will be jealous.	1	3
7.	My partner will be genuinely interested in helping me with my weight.	6	1
8.	I could talk to my partner even if I was doing poorly.	5	1

Getting Support From Others

Picking The Right Person

There are many people who might provide support. Sometimes these people are working on weight control themselves, and you can have a maintenance partnership. Other times, the person may be overweight and may or may not be where you are in terms of weight control, but can still help you with your program. In still other cases, a helping person may not have a weight problem but can understand and support you.

The personal qualities of this person are more important than whether they are heavy, whether they are dieting, how close they live, or whether they are related to you. The Partnership Quiz in this Chapter gives some examples of the qualities to consider in choosing such a person.

Once you have decided you would benefit from support and you know who can be supportive, you need to decide how to start the process. The first step is the realization that most people are not mindreaders. We sometimes expect the people we know to be aware of our needs, to know what to say and when to say it, and how to be supportive at just the right time. Sometimes this happens, but most of the time, reading minds does not work well. You must **make things happen**, not just sit back and wait for people to support you.

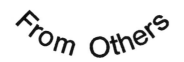

- Ask For Help

- Communicate Openly

- Make Specific Requests

- State Requests Positively

- Reward Your Partner

There are several specific steps you can follow to encourage others to support you. It is important to remember these and to talk these steps over with a person who is working with you.

Ask For Help

Go to a person who might be a supportive helper and ask if they will help. They may be willing, even eager to help, but may not know how to raise the issue or may not know that you would like their help. It is hard for many of us to ask others for help. We think we are imposing or that others will feel pressured to say "yes" when they really mean "stay away, scumball!"

Think about it this way. If a close friend came to you and asked for help, how would you feel? Most of us would feel more than happy to be helpful and would welcome the opportunity to support a friend. Don't your friends feel the same way about you?

Communicate Openly

Speak openly with the person who will be helping you. Talk to them about how you feel and how you would appreciate their help. If talking about your eating and weight is difficult for you, let the person know. Talk about how you would like to be talked to. Should the other person commend you for doing well, be firm when you have trouble, or both? How often should you talk? Would you like the partner to be someone you can **really** talk to, or is a more casual relationship better?

These are important issues, but as we said before, the other person should not have to read your mind. By being open, and by discussing these issues from the very beginning, the partner is in a much better position to help.

Make Specific Requests

As much as possible, give your helping partner **specific** suggestions on how to help. Being vague puts your partner at a disadvantage. As an example, you could say something general like, "Please help me on my program." This is not nearly as helpful as something more specific, such as "Can we walk together every morning at seven?" or "When we go to lunch together, can we go to a place with a salad bar?"

State Requests Positively

We all like to be prodded in a positive way rather than bullied in a negative way. It is human nature. When you are asking a partner for help, there are many ways you can say things. Let's take an example. A woman has trouble when her husband eats ice cream in front of her in the late evening. She could ask him to do this less using a negative approach. She might say, "You are being mean when you eat ice cream in front of me." Or, she could ask for the same change in a positive way by saying, "I would appreciate it if you tried to eat ice cream less in front of me. It would be a big help." Think of things you would like your partner to do, then think of a positive way to ask.

Reward Your Partner

The person who is helping you is going out of their way to be supportive. They are probably happy to do it and expect nothing in return. Nevertheless, we all like to be rewarded. Lasting, satisfying relationships occur when there is equal give and take. If your partner is giving to you, give something in return. You can say a few kind words, pat the person on the back, write a nice note, send flowers, take the person to a movie, get them a gift, or do the dozens of nice things people can do for each other. If the helping person is your romantic partner, a hug, kiss, or even some */&!#@+* might be helpful!

How Much Is Enough?

Some people believe that they should not have to rely on others to control their weight. This feeling is guided by the philosophy that successful maintainers are ones who can do it on their own. In support of this notion, one of us (JR) did a study on people who had successfully maintained weight loss. Some of the people made a special point that they had tapered their reliance on others and were confident they could be successful by themselves.

It is true that the ultimate effort to maintain your weight must come from you. You must decide whether the support you get from others is a helpful boost or a source of dependence. If others are used as a crutch, then you should decide when to begin tapering your reliance on them. Ultimately, you want to attribute your success to yourself and to know that your efforts made the difference. Relying on others is fine as you are getting started, but as time goes on, try to strike a happy balance between needing others and using their help to occasionally give you a needed boost.

A Final Note For Solo Maintainers

We want to emphasize again that solo and social maintainers are different, not better or worse from one another. Some people even switch back and forth from being solo and social. Many individuals go through stages with their weight. At one point, they do not want or need support from others, but then a time might arrive when the social approach is useful. Even if you consider yourself a solo maintainer, you may not always be that way. If a time comes when you feel others could be helpful, refer back to this chapter.

Summary

Support from other people can make a world of difference to some individuals. Look back over the Social vs. Solo Inventory to see if you are a social or a solo maintainer. Once you make this distinction, you can decide the role that support can play in your program. It is important to remember that if you need and want support, it will not leap out at you. You must identify the people who can give it to you and then work to make it happen. It is helpful to remember that support is like a precious mineral lying beneath the ground. If you know how to get it, and then make the effort, it is yours. Waiting around for it to come to you in just the ways you need and want, is like expecting people from the Internal Revenue Service to be graduates of charm school.

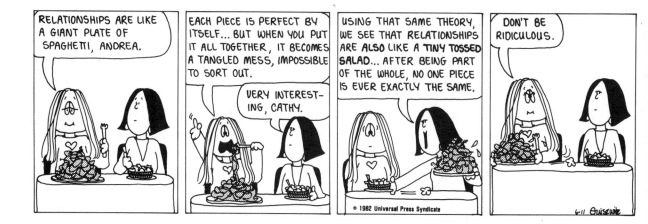

CHAPTER ELEVEN

Anchors A'Weigh

To paraphrase the old Navy song "Anchors Away," your weight should not be what keeps your ship from moving along. Your weight can be another positive component of your maintenance strategy.

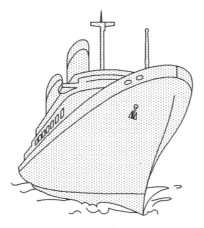

To Weigh or Not to Weigh

People are often confused about how frequently to weigh themselves. Some programs and diet books even recommend not weighing at all.

For maintenance, weighing yourself **is** important. You must use the information differently than when you lose weight, however. Your weight is neither your enemy nor the final goal. It's simply information. Weighing is another diagnostic tool like your food diary, or risk assessment chart. So, the answer to the question of whether to weigh or not is a definite "yes".

How often to weigh depends on you. The important thing is to have a set of guidelines for when to weigh yourself, whether it's every day, once a week, twice a month or whatever. People who have difficulty with maintenance do not have a set of guidelines for deciding when to weigh themselves. They weigh themselves whenever they remember or feel like it. They do not plan for it or think about it ahead of time.

No matter how often you decide to weigh yourself, you must do it at the same time of day each time. Weight fluctuates dramatically throughout the day as the hormones that regulate our biological clock change. Weight also changes with factors such as how much salt we've eaten, how much water we've drunk and other dietary factors. Pick a particular time and stick to it, and certainly do not get weighed more than once a day.

The virtue of weighing frequently (like everyday) is that you get frequent feedback about how you are doing. However, daily fluctuations in weight caused by fluid changes and other factors drive some people crazy. Weighing once a week decreases this problem, but may or may not be frequent enough for you. Think about how often **you** should weigh yourself, then follow through consistently.

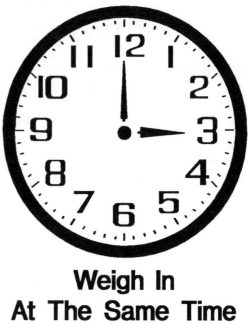

Weigh In
At The Same Time
Each Day

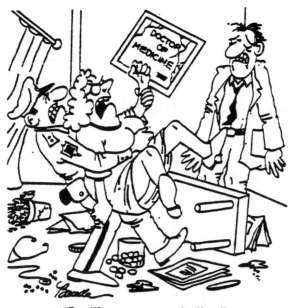

"I still say your scale lies!"

Keeping to Your Weight Goal

We talked in Lesson 2 about choosing a realistic weight target. Remember this is a weight that lets you feel comfortable and good about how you look. In this chapter, we want to help you find a strategy for making that goal work. First, answer the following set of questions about what you are currently doing.

Weight Strategy Questionnaire

Which of the following describes your strategy for keeping yourself at your realistic weight? Remember this is the weight at which you would feel comfortable and feel good about how you look. Please read all six statements and choose only one.

_____   My strategy is to keep my weight at a precise number (e.g. 165 pounds, 125 pounds).

What is that weight? _____ lbs.

_____   My strategy is to keep my weight within a definite range (e.g. 165-167 pounds, 125-135 pounds).

What is your low point on that range? _____ lbs.
What is your high point on that range?_____ lbs.

_____   My strategy is to keep myself within a particular size or set of clothes.

_____   My strategy is to keep myself in a desired shape.

_____   My strategy is different from any of these. It is

_____

_____

_____   I do not have a specific strategy for keeping myself at my realistic weight.

To be a successful maintainer, you must have a specific strategy for keeping yourself at a realistic weight. One strategy is not necessarily better than the others. What is important is to use your strategy **consistently**. By using this strategy, you should feel in control of your weight because you can identify and diagnose when you have run into trouble. Then use the principles covered in the other lessons for getting yourself out of trouble.

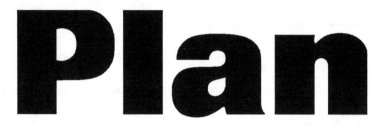

To make sure you are implementing those principles properly, use the questionnaire on the following page. Diagnose how you respond when you find yourself exceeding your planned weight or body size guidelines.

If you find that you are still "very likely" or "extremely likely" to use problem responses like binging, feeling like giving up, getting depressed, or feeling like a failure, it is time to go back and rehearse some of the strategies we already discussed.

If you are at least "somewhat likely" to use more positive, helpful strategies such as increasing your physical activity, restricting your overall food intake, or weighing yourself more frequently, then you are on the road to successful maintenance. Remember that these strategies are only to be implemented when your weight or size goal is surpassed. They are **not** general recommendations for how you should be leading your day-to-day life.

cathy®   **by Cathy Guisewite**

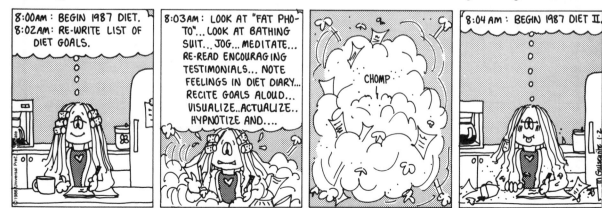

Strategy Implementation Questionaire

When you gain more weight than you want to, how likely are you to:

	Not At All	Not Very	Somewhat	Very Likely	Extremely
Use your food diaries	___	___	___	___	___
Increase your physical activity	___	___	___	___	___
Restrict overall food intake	___	___	___	___	___
Weigh yourself more frequently	___	___	___	___	___
Eliminate snacking	___	___	___	___	___
Eliminate favorite high calorie foods	___	___	___	___	___
Ask other people for help	___	___	___	___	___
Ignore your weight increase	___	___	___	___	___
Increase binging	___	___	___	___	___
Feel like giving up	___	___	___	___	___

In the spaces below, note the most important things **you** can do when you gain weight or when you find yourself struggling for control.

1. _____

2. _____

3. _____

4. _____

5. _____

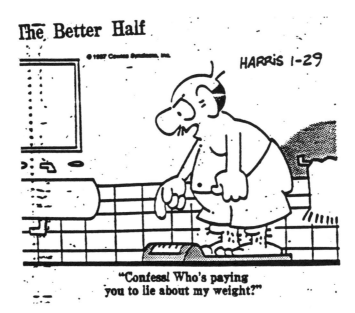

CHAPTER TWELVE

Your Personal Maintenance Check-up

A Maintenance Check-Up Schedule

Earlier in this book (in Chapter 5), we introduced the topic of check-ups. Having regular assessments of your eating, exercise, and attitudes is central to weight maintenance. Your car runs better if you have it checked regularly, and your health will be better if you have periodic medical exams. The same principle applies to your eating and weight.

By making regular assessments of your maintenance strategies, you will accomplish several things. Perhaps most important is that you can spot trouble brewing. You will discover **whether** problems are beginning to occur. Little things may change, and you may not notice. These might be the early warning signs of something worse to come. If you intervene early, the battle is won, but letting things go too far can create a negative momentum that is difficult to break.

Regular check-ups can also tell you **where** the problems exist. Is it your attitudes, your exercise patterns, your eating, your lack of preplanning? This will permit you to target specific problems uncovered by a check-up. You can then refer back to the materials covered in this book that focus on the particular "trouble zone" you have identified.

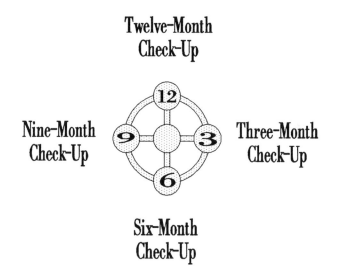

Twelve-Month
Check-Up

Nine-Month
Check-Up

Three-Month
Check-Up

Six-Month
Check-Up

A Schedule For You

The schedule which follows shows how you can keep alert by having a check-up every three months. Mark your calendar now. Three months from today, make a note on your calendar to do your "Three-Month Check-Up." Six months from today, make a note for your "Six-Month Check-Up." Then do the same thing for nine months and twelve months.

We recommend that you follow the check-up schedule for the next two years, and then reevaluate whether you need to continue beyond that. Since each check-up should take less than 30 minutes, and because you are dealing with such an important issue in your life, the burden of doing the check-ups is minimal, and the payoff is great.

Your Personal Maintenance Kit

We realize that it is easiest to do your regular check-ups if the forms are handy and readily accessible. We have, therefore, prepared a **Personal Maintenance Kit** that contains all the forms necessary for each regular check-up for the next two years. This kit contains a detailed description and rationale for the check-ups, a check-up schedule, and the appropriate forms. It is designed to be handy and to save you the trouble of copying all the forms from this book. This kit can be obtained using the ordering information at the end of this book.

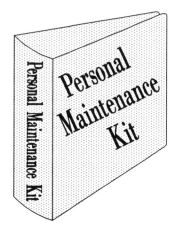

Your Personal Check-Up Schedule

MONTH 3

- ☐ Weight Attitudes Test (questions 5-8 from Maintenance History Questionnaire) (Chapter 1)
- ☐ Control Quiz (Chapter 3)
- ☐ Risk Record (complete for 7 days) (Chapter 3)
- ☐ Preplanning Techniques (Chapter 4)
- ☐ Weight Strategy Questionnaire (Chapter 11)

MONTH 6

- ☐ What I like About Me Scale (Chapter 1)
- ☐ Body Image Exercise (Chapter 2)
- ☐ Feelings About Your Body (Chapter 2)
- ☐ Eating Risk Factors (Chapter 3)
- ☐ Food Diary (complete for 7 days) (Chapter 5)
- ☐ Eating Habits Checklist (Chapter 6)
- ☐ Exercise Quiz (Chapter 7)
- ☐ Strategy Implementation Questionnaire (Chapter 11)

MONTH 9

- ☐ Weight Attitudes Test (questions 5-8 from Maintenance History Questionnaire) (Chapter 1)
- ☐ Control Quiz (Chapter 3)
- ☐ Risk Record (complete for 7 days) (Chapter 3)
- ☐ Preplanning Techniques (Chapter 4)
- ☐ Weight Strategy Questionnaire (Chapter 11)

MONTH 12

- ☐ What I Like About Me Scale (Chapter 1)
- ☐ Body Image Exercise (Chapter 2)
- ☐ Feelings About Your Body (Chapter 2)
- ☐ Eating Risk Factors (Chapter 3)
- ☐ Food Diary (complete for 7 days) (Chapter 5)
- ☐ Eating Habits Checklist (Chapter 6)
- ☐ Exercise Quiz (Chapter 7)
- ☐ Strategy Implementation Questionnaire (Chapter 11)

Consider using the **Personal Maintenance Kit**, even if you now feel confident that you are firmly in control of your eating and weight. Your control may be firm, but periodic check-ups are essential, especially in the first two years after completing a maintenance program. This is when the most lapses are likely to occur. If you do not develop a problem, the kit can reinforce how well you are doing and can show you how much progress you have made. For people who run into trouble, the kit can show when problems arise before they become serious, and perhaps before a person is willing to own up to the fact that trouble is on the way.

Instructions

If you obtain the **Personal Maintenance Kit**, all the items contained here, including the Personal Check-Up Schedule and the instructions for each questionnaire, are contained in the kit. It is a stand-alone kit, with all the necessary information and materials. If you wish to use the forms available in this book, you can reuse or copy the forms from the relevant chapters to make your own kit.

The first step is to use the Personal Check-Up Schedule provided in this section. This schedule shows which chapter each questionnaire comes from, so refer back to that chapter for instructions. After you fill out a questionnaire, use the guidelines that follow for scoring. The guidelines also give you tips about how to react depending on your scores.

Weight Attitudes Test (Chapter 1)

The Weight Attitudes Test includes questions 5-8 of the Maintenance History Questionnaire found in Chapter 1. Complete these 4 questions.

If you checked "Frequently" or "Almost Always" for any of the questions, the diet mentality of breaking rules and feeling guilty is still lurking around. One object of your maintenance effort is to live free of guilt and to devote **less** attention to food and weight.

Read back over Chapter 2 on body weight and body image. Setting reasonable goals and defining a reasonable weight and shape for **you** is one key to feeling satisfied. Also, Chapter 9, on the power of positive thinking, can help with the attitudes that set the stage for guilt. You want to be vigilant, but not obsessive. You want to pay attention to your weight, but not let it govern your life.

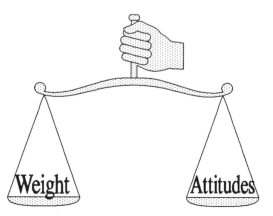

Control Quiz (Chapter 3)

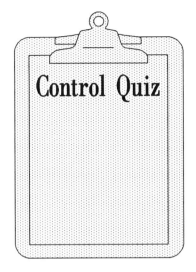

The Control Quiz strikes at the very core of how you feel about eating and weight. In many cases, **feeling** vulnerable makes a person **be** more vulnerable. The Control Quiz distinguishes control over eating and control over weight. Question 1 deals with weight and the remaining questions deal with eating.

Think of how you completed the quiz when you were just beginning the program, and see how your responses have changed. The goal is for you to score in the middle of the range of answers. For example, if you circled "Slightly" or "Somewhat" to question 1, you have some fear about regaining weight, but the fear is under control. Higher scores reflect lingering doubts you might have about your ability to maintain.

If you score higher than in the middle range, Chapters 3 and 4, which deal with Risk Assessment and Relapse Prevention, will be particularly helpful. Go back and read this information and plan out specific ideas for giving yourself better control. This will help you feel less vulnerable.

Risk Record (Chapter 3)

The Risk Record is to be filled out for 7 days. Make seven copies of the form in Chapter 3, or if you have the **Personal Maintenance Kit**, the copies are provided for you. The Risk Record helps you identify the situations, feelings, times, and places associated with high-risk situations.

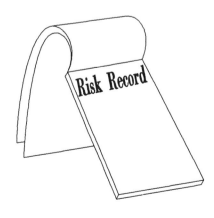

After completing the Risk Record for seven days, you can reflect back on how you completed the form initially. Have your risk situations changed? It is important to be honest with yourself about when you feel you are at risk. Even if you don't overeat or gain weight, you might still feel at risk. The Risk Record will help you specify what puts you at risk. Then you can use the information in Chapters 3 and 4 to follow one of two paths: avoid the risk, or cope with the risk.

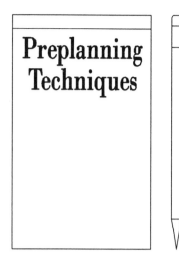

Preplanning Techniques (Chapter 4)

The information that you collect from the Risk Record can now be used to complete your list of preplanning techniques. This is a list that you will store in your memory, so you will know exactly what to do when you encounter a high-risk situation.

Write down your high-risk situations on the left side of the form. To the right of each situation, fill in the line labeled "What I Will Do." As you are filling these in, think of concrete actions you can take to remove you from the risk, remove risk from the situation, or respond to risk when you encounter it.

Weight Strategy Questionnaire (Chapter 11)

One thing that characterizes successful maintainers is that they tend to have a specific weight strategy. They define a weight they want to maintain, or more often, have a weight **range** they will maintain. Others want to remain in a given size of clothing or want to be a certain shape.

Successful maintainers know exactly how they will respond if they violate their weight strategy. One person, for example, might reread this book if weight goes above a certain level. Another might join a local weight loss program when clothes do not fit.

Use this questionnaire to note which maintenance strategy you will use. It is important to have a strategy, even though different people might use different approaches. Most important is to know **what** you will do if the alarm sounds and you need to take corrective action.

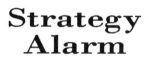

Strategy Alarm

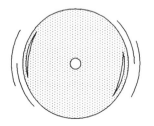

What I Like About Me Scale (Chapter 1)

This scale is your way of feeling good about your good qualities. There are many aspects to being a good human being, and too often people let their weight dominate how they feel about the rest of their lives. It is important to keep weight in perspective. If you are not satisfied with how you look, read Chapter 2 about reasonable goals and establishing a realistic weight and shape. If you still feel dissatisfied, think about how you can put it in perspective by feeling good about your other qualities.

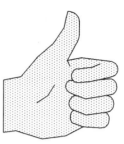

What I Like About Me Scale

Body Image Exercise (Chapter 2)

Use the silhouettes provided in Chapter 2 to rate how you feel you look and how you would like to look. The instructions for doing this appear with the figures.

If there is a discrepancy between how you feel you look and how you would like to look, ask yourself several questions. First, would other people rate you the way you rate yourself? If you rate yourself as heavier than others would, then your perceptions and feelings about yourself may be unrealistic. Many people who have lost weight still feel heavy. This feeling can be a problem because it leads to never feeling satisfied.

The second important question is whether your desired weight is reasonable. If you aspire to a weight or shape that is not possible for you to attain, you are racing headlong into a stone wall. Use the information in Chapter 2 on selecting a reasonable weight and shape.

Body Image Exercise

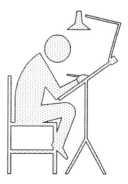

Feelings About Your Body (Chapter 2)

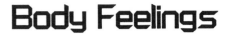

This scale is a rating of how you feel about your body weight and shape. Use the instructions that accompany the scale in Chapter 2 to give a 1-7 rating for your feelings about each part of your body.

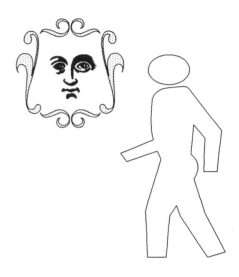

One objective of a good weight management program is to help people accept, enjoy, and derive pleasure from their bodies. This can happen even when people do not lose weight, or when they regain what they have lost. Our bodies are part of us, and it is a tragedy for people to dislike this important part of their being.

Compare your answers on this scale to your earlier answers. Are you showing positive changes? Do you now accept your body and feel like it can be a positive part of your life? Chapter 2 provides useful information on making this happen.

Eating Risk Factors (Chapter 3)

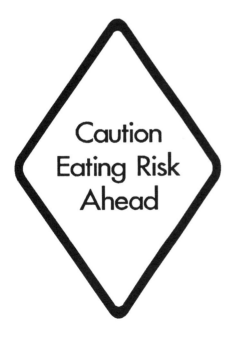

This form permits you to identify the aspects of different situations that place you at risk. Fill out this form and think carefully about what makes a situation risky for you.

An example of a typical response on this form might be as follows. One person finds driving home from work risky because he stops in the drive-in window of a fast food restaurant. The risk may be created by hunger (he has not eaten since noon), fatigue, or frustration with work.

Knowing what creates risk is the first step in controlling risk. Using the above example, the man could pack a small salad and then eat this just before leaving from work. He could listen to relaxing music on the radio. These are several ways he might avoid the risk by first understanding it.

Food Diary (Chapter 5)

Copy and complete the Food Diary for seven days, or if you obtain the **Personal Maintenance Kit**, the copies will be provided for you.

The Food Diary is designed to help you find patterns in your eating. Look for patterns in when you eat, how you eat, and how you feel when you eat. If some patterns are problematic, like eating when bored or tired, you can plan accordingly. The information in Chapter 5 shows which patterns to look for. Chapter 6 then provides suggestions for changing difficult patterns.

Food Diary

Eating Habits Checklist (Chapter 6)

This checklist is designed to help spot problems with binge eating or compulsive eating. Higher scores show there are problems with these eating patterns. Because these patterns can make weight control difficult, it is important to spot them early.

Chapter 6 provides ideas about how to deal with different eating patterns. If you feel you eat compulsively, review this information. If you feel more help is needed, check with various weight programs and health professionals in your community to find someone who can work with you.

Eating Habits
Checklist

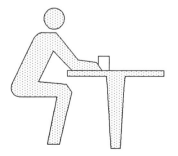

Exercise Quiz (Chapter 7)

As we discussed throughout this book, exercise is one activity that helps a great many people lose weight. One key to exercise is finding a type or types of exercise you like. This varies considerably from person to person, so there is no "best" exercise. Any exercise is good.

The Exercise Quiz will help guide you to the exercise that best suits your personal needs. In addition, it addresses your motivation to exercise. If you find your motivation declining, do something right away. Read over Chapter 7. If it would help, join a club or class so you will have a time and place to exercise. Make a commitment to exercise with a friend. Do whatever it takes to be active.

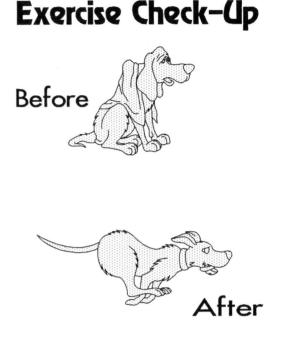

Strategy Implementation Questionnaire (Chapter 11)

When all is said and done about weight control, what matters is whether you have a plan. A plan is something you use when you need help, and even use when you face the day-to-day difficulties that can disrupt your weight control efforts. Being prepared is the key.

The Strategy Implementation Questionnaire permits you to rate the importance of various techniques, so you can then use the ones that are most helpful for you. Have these ready just like you might have a fire extinguisher ready in the house.

In Summary

Having a check-up schedule is important to your weight maintenance efforts. The goal is for you to have a plan, a system, a scheme, a strategy. Call it what you like, but being prepared by having regular check-ups will allow you to nip problems in the bud. It will also show you how many positive changes you have made, and since we all like to be patted on the back, make a vow to yourself right now to follow the check-up schedule we have outlined in this chapter.

Remember:

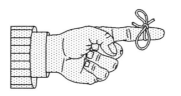

Regular Check-Ups Are Critical To Weight Control

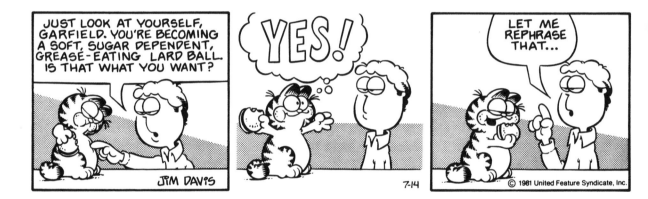

CHAPTER THIRTEEN

Summary: Peering Into Your Future

A Commitment to Permanence

This program began with our commitment to help you maintain weight permanently. This is a lofty goal, but one you **can** reach. The answer lies not in the newest diet book, not in some magic answer the latest talk show guest provides, and not in the alignment of the stars and moon. It lies in the consistency of your own behavior. The goals you set, the way you deal with food and exercise, and the way you think and feel will make the difference.

This book is designed to propel you in the direction of permanent weight control. No matter how strong or weak your confidence and skills might be at this moment, you have laid the foundation for maintenance. You now know how to think, plan, and act to keep weight off. These skills belong to you and are at your disposal when needed. You may need them today, tomorrow, or five years from now, but you can feel good that you know what to do.

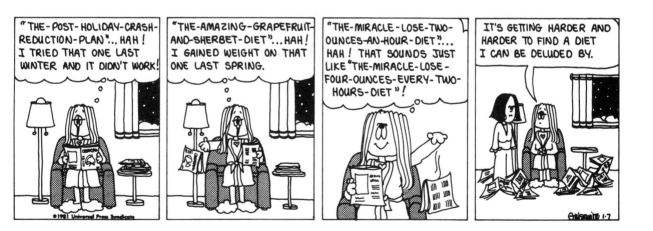

Feeling confident in your abilities involves seeing both the big picture and the small details. In the case of weight maintenance, the big picture is the collection of lifestyle principles you have learned. The details are understanding the ins and outs of **your** eating and exercise patterns, and being aware of how you think and feel. Knowing what to do in a broad sense will permit you to be flexible and then to apply the knowledge when you most need it.

You may learn, for example, to react to mistakes in a constructive rather than negative way. This is the principle. You may apply this to a different situation than another person, but the fact that you **can** apply it shows just how much you have learned.

We would like to emphasize several key points in this final chapter. These represent the core of a maintenance program. Keep these points stored in your memory just like you store your telephone number or social security number. When you need the information, it's there.

Reasonable Weight and Shape

One of the barriers to successful weight maintenance is having unrealistic images of what you can weigh and how you will look. It would be one thing if these images were based in reality, but the cultural ideals of the perfect body are shaped by television and magazine celebrities and models who may be eating next to nothing and exercising compulsively to look the way they do.

You **may** be able to look the way the models do, but then you may not. Even if you could look this way, the key question is whether it is worth the price you must pay. Your genetics, your weight and dieting history, and your feelings about eating and exercise all make a difference in your weight and shape. This is why it is so important to have a **reasonable** weight in mind and to have a realistic image of the body shape you will attain.

We discussed this issue in Chapter 2. Look back over this material and answer the questions we posed to help determine what a realistic weight is for you. In many cases, the realistic weight is different from a person's initial goal, but is still likely to deliver important health benefits and make you feel better about yourself. Keep this weight in your mind, and know how your body will look at that weight, and then feel satisfied when you reach this destination. You may have less than the perfect body, but then who is perfect?

Knowing and Controlling Risk

An insightful person strives to be in situations that lead to good behavior and positive feelings, and avoids situations that create problems. Even though this makes all the sense in the world, it is sometimes difficult to steer away from trouble and even more difficult to always do what we know is best. This is why weight maintenance can be so difficult for some people, and is also why it is so important to understand the concept of risk.

We do many things to avoid risk. We wear seat belts to avoid the risk created by car accidents. We avoid certain areas at night, we look before crossing a street, and we don't swim in shark-infested waters. We know that risk exists, so in these cases are willing to be cautious.

As we discussed in Chapter 3, identifying your risky situations is one of the first steps in successful weight maintenance. We cannot tell you which situations are risky for you, because what is a problem for you may not be a problem for another person. People who maintain their weight know themselves and learn to be sensitive to their own risk.

If you learn to anticipate situations that give you trouble, you can take two actions. The first is to avoid the situations, which if possible, is always a good idea. The second action involves being prepared. You can go a long way toward permanent maintenance if you know in advance how you will handle the situations you are likely to face. In the best of all worlds, you would be totally prepared and would execute your plan no matter what situation you encountered. Because we are human, there may be situations that throw you for a loop no matter how prepared you are. Our goal is to make sure you are prepared for most situations most of the time.

Who Is Responsible Here?

You are. We want to avoid the classic no-win position that many people face when they are struggling with eating and weight.

Here is how it goes for far too many people. A person loses weight and the credit goes to the program. What is the first question people ask when someone has lost weight? "How did you do it"? This implies that the program or approach was the answer. When a person regains some of the weight, do people blame the program? No way. They blame the person. This is the way most people feel about their own weight, and it just isn't fair.

One can get away from this by giving the program all the credit and all the blame. When you lose and maintain, the program is responsible. If a person regains, the program is at fault. This would be more fair, but is wrong.

You are responsible for your eating and weight. Your biology may impose certain limits on how much you weigh and the shape of your body, but beyond this, it is your behavior that counts. This is good news for people who are trying to maintain their weight.

You should feel good about the progress you have made. We may have provided pointers and given you some direction, but it was your decision to change. We did not do it for you. You have a right to feel proud and to know deep inside that you get the credit.

We emphasize this point because of something called attribution theory. This theory shows that people who attribute their behavior to external influences are less likely to maintain the behavior than people who feel the change occurred for internal reasons. For weight control, it is important to give yourself credit where credit is due. If you worked hard to control your weight, the impetus came from you, the effort came from you, and the commitment came from you. Feel good about it and know that it was you who did the changing. This also means that it is you who can keep it going, even when you are finished with the formal materials we have provided in this book.

On Being Human

One key to life is handling imperfection. Some people are frightened by not doing things well, so they don't even try. Others get down on themselves for making mistakes and are always feeling bad. One thing that characterizes successful, happy people is that they accept the fact that they make mistakes and they continue on. They learn from mistakes and try not to repeat them, but they don't feel that each slip in life is a catastrophe.

Many people who are trying to control their weight respond to slips like they would to a catastrophe. They feel terrible, ashamed, and even terrified that the slip signals loss of control. We have emphasized that your response should be logical, calm, and constructive. The object should be to have a reaction ready for any problem you might face, so you can respond by learning and correcting the reason for the problem.

The key to this philosophy is to treat your weight like you would other parts of your life. We all make mistakes. We take the wrong turn while driving, we might slip and say something insensitive, or we do better at work some days than others. We accept these as part of life and move on. We try to figure out what happened and then see that we do better next time. The same approach applies to weight control.

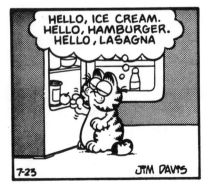 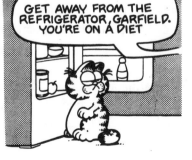 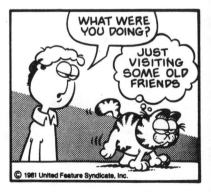

On Being Active

One of the best ways to help maintain your weight is to exercise. People who exercise are more likely to maintain their weight loss than are people who do not. Some scientists believe that exercise lowers the body weight set point (the weight the body wants to maintain). Others believe that exercise stimulates the body to take in healthier foods. We believe the psychological effects of exercise are influential, because people feel better about themselves and are better able to control their eating and weight. Whatever the reasons, exercise helps.

In Chapter 7, we have tried to underscore several key points about exercise. The first is that you don't have to do a lot to benefit. A regular walking program, for example, can help with your weight and may have important health benefits. If you are exercising more often or more vigorously, so much the better, but you can feel good about **any** activity you get.

The second point is that exercise should be fun. Think of ways to make it enjoyable. You might be the type who likes to play tennis with friends. You might like to walk by yourself or watch TV while riding the exercise bike. You might enjoy hiking or swimming or aerobics. If you like it, you will do it, so try to plan out an activity or series of activities that you will enjoy.

Taking Advantage of Resources

There are many resources available for people working to maintain their weight. In Chapter 10, we discussed how support from other people can be a resource. If you feel this is the case for you, that chapter gives guidelines for identifying people who can support you and how to gain their support.

Aside from the help of other people, there are several additional types of resources that you might use. The first is this book. In our experience, this book can be every bit as valuable a year or two from now as it is at this moment. Many people we have worked with keep the book handy and then refer to it either on a regular basis or when needed in a crisis.

Using the book on a regular basis is like having booster shots to develop immunity to a disease. You have an initial shot, but then need periodic boosters to keep your resistance high. You have had the initial shot for weight maintenance by reading this book. To keep your strength and motivation high, you may want to reread the book or parts of the book at regular intervals.

If you used this book as part of an organized program, or along with help from a health professional, consider keeping in touch with the program or professional. Call them for support or advice if you feel you need help or even a little boost. These people can be helpful, either by working with you themselves or by suggesting alternatives.

Another resource comes from weight control programs in your community. A look through the yellow pages will show you many options. In addition to these organized programs, there are professionals such as dietitians, psychologists and fitness specialists who can help. Some people, even those who are successfully maintaining their weight, attend such programs or see a professional because they want or need the continued support. Others initiate such help when they start having trouble, or if they regain a certain number of pounds.

A Check-Up Reminder

In Chapter 12 we emphasized the importance of regular assessments of your eating, weight, behavior, exercise, and attitudes. We have outlined a check-up schedule and also noted that you can obtain the **Personal Maintenance Kit** using the information provided at the end of this book.

Think of yourself as a forest ranger whose job is to protect the forest from fires. The ranger does not wait for a major fire to be underway before taking action. Instead, the ranger makes regular checks of the forest from the tower. This permits immediate action when small fires break out.

By doing regular check-ups, you can spot problems as they begin to develop. This allows you to leap into action and to take decisive steps to get back on the right course. The check-ups are important no matter how confident you are that you will maintain your weight loss. We have a two-year check-up schedule in Chapter 12, so be certain to refer back to this as you complete this book.

Saying Farewell

We enjoyed writing this book and hope you enjoyed reading it. Even more important, however, is our hope that you are on your way to permanent weight maintenance. The necessary skills and attitudes can be yours.

We know how important the issue of weight maintenance is to the people who read this book. We have brought together the latest in what is known in the science of weight control and have merged this with the experience we have with thousands of people in our programs.

We have attempted to make this book a partnership between you and us. We can help bring you the newest and most helpful information, and you can then apply it to your own life. We are confident that you can do it. Even if you are not completely confident that you have a permanent solution, this will come with time. As you practice your new skills and develop techniques to deal with different situations, your confidence will grow. With this comes successful weight maintenance.

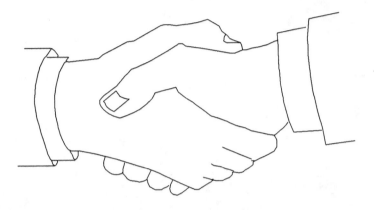

Good Luck!!

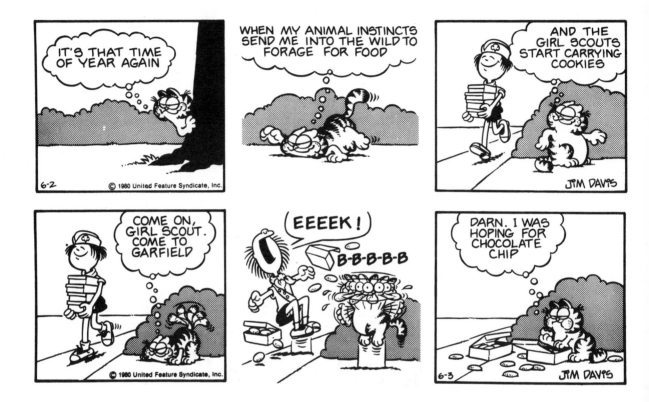

APPENDIX A

The Calorie Guide

This calorie list is condensed from *The Partnership Diet Program*, by K. D. Brownell, published by Rawson-Wade. The values are based on data published in the U.S. Department of Agriculture Handbook No. 465, and by the Smith, Kline, and French Laboratories.

Calories are listed for average serving sizes whenever possible. You may wish to convert some measurements to others to simplify matters. For example, some beverages are listed in fluid ounces while others are listed in cups. Several measurement equivalents are shown below to help with this task.

1 cup = 8 fluid ounces   1 cup = 1/2 pint

1 cup = 16 tablespoons   2 tabelspoons = 1 fluid ounce

1 tablespoon = 3 teaspoons   1 quart = 4 cups

1 pound = 16 ounces

Alcohol (see Beverages)		Apricots	
Almonds		raw, 3 medium	55
shelled, 1 cup	849	canned in water, 1 cup	93
chopped, 1 cup	777	canned in syrup, 1 cup	222
roasted (in oil), 1 oz	178	dried, uncooked, 1 cup	338
Anchovy, 1 oz	49	Artichoke, globe, cooked	53
Apples		Artichoke hearts, 3 frozen	22
1 raw with skin, 3 in diam.	96	Asparagus	
1 baked with 2 tbsp sugar	172	raw, 5-6 spears	26
Apple butter, 1 tbsp	33	cooked, 4 spears	12
Apple juice, 1 cup	117	canned, 1 cup spears	94
Apple sauce		Avocado, 1 medium	378
unsweetened, 1 cup	100	Bacon	
sweetened, 1 cup	232	cooked, 2 slices	86

Canadian, 1 slice cooked	58	cider, 4 oz	125
Bagel, 1 water	55	cocoa, with milk, 1 cup	175
Baking powder, 1 tbsp	14	coffee (1 cup)	
Bamboo shoots, 1 cup	40	black	5
Banana, 1 medium	101	with sugar	35
Barbecue sauce, 1 cup	228	with sugar & cream	65
Bass		lemonade, 8 oz	105
baked, stuffed, 1 oz	73	milk (8 oz)	
oven fried, 1 oz	56	chocolate	205
Beans (1 cup cooked)		skim	80
green	31	whole	160
kidney	218	milk shake, 8 oz	420
lima	189	soft drinks (12 oz)	
navy	224	cola	144
northern	212	cream soda	156
yellow	28	fruit drinks	168
Bean sprouts, 1 cup raw	45	ginger ale	109
Beans and franks, 1 cup	367	root beer	156
Beef (cooked, 4 oz)		tea (1 cup)	
brisket, lean	253	no sugar	0
chuck for stew, lean	243	with sugar	30
chuck, ground, lean	315	with sugar & milk	40
chuck roast, lean	219	Beverages (alcoholic)	
club steak, lean	278	beer and ale	
flank steak, lean	222	ale, 8 oz	100
ground, regular	324	beer, regular, 12 oz	156
ground, lean	248	beer, light, 12 oz	104
porterhouse steak	255	distilled spirits	
rib roast, lean	275	brandy, 1 pony glass	70
round steak, lean	214	cognac, 1 pony glass	70
sirloin steak, lean	235	gin, 100 proof, 1 jigger	124
T-bone steak, lean	253	rum, 100 proof, 1 jigger	124
Beef, corned		vodka, 100 proof, 1 jigger	124
boiled, 4 oz	424	whiskey, 1 jigger	110
canned, 4 oz	245	liqueurs and cordials (1 oz)	
hash, 4 oz	231	absinthe	84
Beef, chipped, creamed, 1 cup	420	anisette	111
Beef stew, 4 oz	90	Benedictine	112
Beer (see Beverages)		brandy, fruit	86
Beets		Cherry Heering	80
cooked, 2	32	creme de menthe	110
canned, 1 cup	63	Drambuie	110
Beverages (nonalcoholic)		Southern Comfort	120

triple sec	83		Breadcrumbs, 1 cup	392
mixed drinks			Bread pudding, 1 cup	496
daiquiri, 3.5 oz	120		Bread sticks, 5 large	192
highball, 4 oz	83		Bread stuffing, 1 cup	416
Manhattan, 3.5 oz	165		Broccoli	
martini, 3.5 oz	140		raw, 3 stalks (1 lb)	145
old fashioned, 4 oz	180		cooked, 1 stalk	47
Tom Collins, 10 oz	180		Brussels sprouts, 1 cup	56
wines (4 oz)			Buns	
Beaujolais	96		cinnamon, 1	160
Bordeaux	96		hot cross, 1	110
Burgundy	96		Butter	
champagne	108		regular, 1 tbsp	102
Chianti	100		whipped, 1 tbsp	67
liebfraumilch	84			
port	184			
Rhine	96			
Riesling	90		Cabbage, cooked, 1 cup	29
rose	95		Cakes (1/12 of cake)	
sherry, cream	200		angel food	161
vermouth, Italian	189		Boston cream pie	311
Biscuits, 1 medium	130		coffee cake	195
Blackberries, 1 cup	85		cupcake	172
Blueberries, 1 cup	85		devils food	443
Bluefish, broiled, 4 oz	120		fruit cake	163
Bologna (see sausage)			gingerbread	371
Bouillon, 1 cube	5		layer	310
Brains, raw, 3 oz	105		pound	142
Bran, 1 cup	120		spice	363
Branflakes, 1 cup	106		white	390
Braunschweiger (see sausage)			yellow	365
Breads (1 slice or piece)			Cake icing, 1/2 cup	620
banana	135		Candy	
corn	95		butterscotch, 1 piece	20
French	44		candy corn, 10 pieces	51
hoagie or submarine roll	392		caramel, 1 piece	43
Italian	83		chocolate	
protein	45		semisweet, 1 oz	144
pumpernickel	80		milk, 1 oz	147
raisin	66		bar, 2 oz	300
rye	55		kisses, 1 oz	150
white	74		fudge, 1 oz	113
whole wheat	56		gumdrops, 8 small	35

hard, 1 piece	3	Wheat Chex, 1/2 cup	100
Hershey milk, 1-1/2 oz	210	Wheaties	105
jellybeans, 10	104	Cheese (1 oz)	
lollipop, 1 large	215	American	105
Mars bar, 1 oz	160	blue	104
Mars Milky Way, 1 oz	120	Camembert, domestic	84
Mars 3 Musketeers, 1 oz	120	Cheddar	111
marshmallows, 1 regular	23	cottage	30
peanut brittle, 1 oz	119	cottage, 1/2 cup	120
Cantaloupe, 1/2 melon	60	cream	106
Carrots		Edam	105
raw, 1	30	Gorgonzola	112
cooked, 1 cup	48	Gouda	108
Cashew nuts, 9 medium	80	Gruyere	115
Catfish, 3.5 oz	105	Limburger	98
Catsup (see ketchup)		Monterey	102
Cauliflower, 1 cup	28	mozzarella	79
Caviar, 1 tbsp	42	muenster	100
Celery, 1 stalk	7	Parmesan	110
Cereals (1 cup)		Parmesan, 1 tbsp	29
All Bran	192	provolone	99
Alpha Bits	110	Romano	110
branflakes	106	Romano, grated, 1 tbsp	30
Cap'n Crunch	151	Roquefort	110
Cheerios	89	Swiss	104
Cocoa Krispies	113	Velveeta	90
corn flakes	95	Cheese Twists, 5 pieces	16
Cream of Wheat	130	Cherries, sour red, 1 cup	90
farina	140	Chewing gum, 1 piece	5
Grape Nuts, 1/4 cup	110	Chicken	
Kellogg's Special K	60	broiled, 4 oz	154
Kix	100	fried, breast, 1	160
Lucky Charms	97	fried, thigh, 1	122
Maypo, 3/4 cup	115	roasted, no skin, 4 oz	207
oatmeal	150	Chicken a la King, 1 cup	468
puffed rice	50	Chicken fricassee, 1 cup	368
Product 19	110	Chicken pot pie, small pie	545
Rice Krispies	105	Chickpeas, raw, 1 cup	720
shredded wheat, 1 oz	85	Chili con carne	
Sugar Frosted Flakes	143	with beans, 1 cup	339
Sugar Pops	110	without beans, 1 cup	512
Sugar Smacks	110	Chili powder, 1 tbsp	51
Trix	112	Chocolate (see candy)	

Chocolate syrup

light type, 1 tbsp	23
fudge type, 1 tbsp	62
Chop suey, 1 cup	300
Chow mein, chicken, 1 cup	255

Cider (see beverages)

Clams

cherrystone, 6 large	56
steamers, 4 large, 9 small	80
Clam dip, sour cream,1 tsp	8

Cocoa (see beverages)

Coconut, shredded, 1 cup	345
Codfish, broiled, 4 oz	192

Coffee (see beverages)

Cola (see beverages)

Cold cuts (see sausage)

Coleslaw, 1 cup	155
Collards, cooked, 1 cup	59

Cookies

Animal Crackers	10
applesauce	33
brownies, nuts, not iced	97
butter	23
chocolate chip	50
chocolate fudge sandwich	100
creme sandwich	46
fig bar	50
gingersnaps	30
graham cracker	30
macaroon	90
molasses	137
oatmeal, with raisins	59
Oreo	40
peanut butter	55
sugar	36
sugar wafers	46
vanilla wafer	19

Cooking oil (see oils)

Corn

cooked, 1 ear	70
cooked, 1 cup	137

Cornbread (see breads)

Corn muffins (see muffins)

Corn oil (see oil)

Cornstarch, 1 tbsp	30

Cornsyrup (see syrup)

Cottage cheese (see cheese)

Crab

canned, 4 oz	116
cooked (steamed), 4 oz	55

Crackers

animal	12
cheese	15
graham	30
matzo	80
Melba toast	15
oyster	3
Ritz	15
Ry-Krisp	20
saltine	15
soda	30
Triscuit	20
Wheat Thins	10
Zwieback	30
Cranberries, raw, 1 cup	44
Cranberry juice, 6 oz	124
Cranberry sauce, 1 cup	404

Cream

half & half, 1 tbsp	20
light, 1/2 cup	253
light, 1 tbsp	32
heavy, 2 cups whipped	838
sour, 1 cup	455
sour, 1 tbsp	29
Cream puff, 1	303
Cucumber, 1 medium	15
Custard, baked, 1 cup	305
Dates, pitted, 10	219

Deviled ham (see sausage)

Dips (1 oz)

bacon	71
blue cheese	69
clam	67
onion	70

Donuts

cake	125

jelly	225	Gingerbread (see cakes)	
raised or yeast	125	Ginger root, fresh, 1 oz	14
sugared or iced	150	Grapefruit, 1/2 medium	40
Duck, roasted, 1 slice	110	Grapefruit juice, 1 cup	96
		Grapes, 10 concord	18
Eggs		Grape drink, 1 cup	135
		Grape juice, 1 cup	167
fresh, 1 large	82	Gravy (1/2 cup)	
fresh, whites, 1	17	beef	60
fresh, yolks, 1	59	chicken	108
fried, 1 large	99	mushroom	60
poached, 1 large	82	Gum (see chewing gum)	
scrambled, 1 large	111	Haddock, fried, 4 oz	188
Eggnog (see beverages)		Halibut, broiled, 4 oz	172
Eggplant, cooked, 1 cup	38	Ham (see pork)	
Escarole, 7 small leaves	5	Hamburger (see beef)	
Farina (see cereals)		Hash, corned beef (see beef)	
Figs, 1 medium	40	Herbs	0
Fish (see individual kinds)		Herring, pickled, 1 oz	63
Fish cakes, fried, 4 oz	195	Hollandaise sauce, 1/2 cup	59
Fish sticks, 1 stick	50	Honey, 1 tbsp	64
Flounder, 1 oz	57	Honeydew (see muskmelon)	
Flour		Horseradish, 1 oz	18
enriched, 1 cup	450	Ice cream (1/3 pint)	
wheat, 1 cup sifted	400	chocolate	191
Frankfurters (see sausage)		strawberry	174
French toast, 1 slice	185	vanilla	180
Frog legs, 6 large	420	French, vanilla	247
Frostings (see cake icing)		frozen custard, 1 cup	334
Frozen custard (see ice cream)		sherbet, orange	152
Fruit (see individual listing)		Ice cream bar, 3 oz	150
Fruit cocktail		Ice cream cone, waffle	19
water pack, 1 cup	91	Ice cream sandwich	208
syrup pack, 1 cup	194	Ice cream soda, 8 oz	255
Garbanzos (see chickpeas)		Ice milk, vanilla, 1/3 pint	135
Garlic, raw, 1 clove	4	Ice milk bar	144
Gelatin		Icings (see cake icings)	
plain, 1 tablespoon	35	Jams, 1 tbsp	54
fruit flavors, 1/2 cup	80	Jellies, 1 tbsp	55
fruit flavors, 1 square	140	Juice (see types)	
diet, 1/2 cup	8	Kale, raw, 4 oz	80
Gin (see beverages)		Ketchup, 1 tbsp	20
Ginger ale (see beverages)		Knockwurst (see sausage)	

Lamb	
leg, 4 oz	211
loin chops, lean, 4 oz	213
Lard, 1 tbsp	117
Leeks, raw, 1	17
Lemon, peeled,	20
Lemonade, 6 oz	81
Lemon juice, 1 tbsp	4
Lentils, cooked, 1 cup	212
Lettuce (fresh)	
iceberg, 1 head	70
iceberg, 3 leaves	6
romaine, 1 cup	10
Lima beans (see beans)	
Limes, 1	19
Liver (cooked)	
beef, 4 oz	260
chicken, 4 oz	187
Liverwurst, (see sausage)	
Lobster, cooked, 1 cup	138
Lobster Newberg, 1 cup	485
Lox, 4 oz	200
Luncheon meats (see sausage)	
Macadamia nuts, 6	106
Macaroni	
cooked, 2 1/5 cups	419
cooked, 1 cup	155
Macaroni & cheese, 1 cup	430
Mackerel, broiled, 4 oz	248
Mangoes, 1 fruit	152
Margarine	
1 stick, 4 oz	816
1 pat	36
1 tbsp	102
Marshmallow (see candy)	
Mayonnaise (see salad dressing)	
Meatloaf (see sausage)	
Meats (see beef, lamb, pork)	
Melba toast, 1 slice	25
Melons (see types)	
Milk, cow (1 cup)	
whole (3.5% fat)	159
skim	88

low fat (2% fat)	145
dry, regular	643
dry, instant	351
dry, nonfat, regular	436
dry, nonfat, instant	80
Milk shake (see beverages)	
Molasses, 1 tbsp	46
Muffins	
plain	118
blueberry	112
bran	104
corn	126
Mushrooms, sliced, 1 cup	20
Muskmelons (1/2 melon)	
cantaloupe	60
casaba	184
honeydew	248
Mussels, 4 oz	108
Mustard, 1 tsp	5
Mutton (see lamb)	
Nectarine	88
Noodles	
egg, cooked, 1 cup	200
chow mein, canned, 1 cup	220
Nuts (see individual kinds)	
Nuts, mixed, 8-12	95
Oatmeal (see cereal)	
Ocean perch, fried, 4 oz	256
Oils, all vegetable, 1 tbsp	120
Okra, sliced, 1 cup	36
Olives, 5 small	16
Omelet (see eggs)	
Onions	40
Onion rings, frozen, 4 oz	146
Oranges	71
Orange juice, 1 cup	120
Oysters, (13-19 medium)	158
Pancakes, 1 large	164
Papaya, medium	119
Parsley, 10 sprigs	4
Parsnips, raw, 1/2 lb	146
Pastina, 1 cup	651
Pastries	

cream puff	303	Pistachios, shelled, 1/4 lb	674
Danish, 1 small	150	Pizza (1/8 of 14 in. pie)	
Peaches		cheese	153
medium, 1	38	sausage & cheese	157
canned, water pack, 1 cup	76	Plums	
Peanuts, 10 nuts	105	prune type, 1	21
Peanut butter, 1 tbsp	94	canned, water pack, 1 cup	114
Pears		Pomegranate, 1 medium	97
medium, 1	100	Popcorn	
canned, water pack, 1 cup	78	popped, plain, 1 cup	23
Peas, black-eyed (see cowpeas)		popped in oil, 1 cup	41
Peas, 1/2 cup		Popovers, 1 medium	60
boiled	57	Pork (4 oz)	
canned	82	bacon (see bacon)	
frozen	69	ham, boiled	266
Pecans, 10 medium	96	ham, roasted	426
Peppers, sweet, 1 cup	18	ham, deviled	398
Perch (see ocean perch)		loin roast, lean	288
Pickles		loin chops, lean	302
dill, 1 medium	7	spareribs, braised	500
sweet, Gherkins, 1	22	Pork and beans, 1/2 cup	160
relish, sweet, 1 tbsp.	21	Potatoes	
Pies (baked, 4 3/4 in.arc)		baked, 1 medium	145
apple	404	French fried, 4 oz	311
banana cream	350	French fried, 10 strips	200
blueberry	382	fried, 1 cup	456
Boston cream (see cakes)		hashed brown, 1 cup	355
butterscotch	406	mashed, with milk, 1 cup	137
cherry	412	scalloped, 1 cup	355
chocolate meringue	383	sweet potatoes, 4 oz	125
custard	331	Potato chips	
lemon meringue	357	10 chips	114
mince	428	1 oz	161
pecan	577	Potato salad, 1 cup	248
pumpkin	321	Pretzels	
shoo-fly	440	Dutch, 1 large	60
sweet potato	324	10 sticks or 1 three-ring	10
Pie crust, 1 pie shell	900	Prunes, dried, 1 cup	253
Pike, 4 oz.	102	Prune juice, 1 cup	197
Pineapple		Puddings (1/2 cup)	
fresh, diced, 1 cup	81	banana	165
canned, water pack, 1 cup	96	butterscotch	190
Pineapple juice, 1 cup	138	chocolate	190

custard	145	Thousand Island		80
rice	140	Thousand Island, diet		27
tapioca, vanilla	170	vinegar and oil		65
vanilla	165	Salad oil (see oils)		
Pumpkin, canned, 1 cup	81	Salads		
Pumpkin seeds, 1/2 cup	387	apple-carrot, 1/2 cup		100
Quail, 4 oz	172	carrot-raisin, 3 tbsp		155
Quinces, 4 oz	79	coleslaw (see coleslaw)		
Rabbit, 4 oz	245	chicken & celery, 3 tbsp		180
Radishes, 10 medium	8	comb. vegetable, 1 cup		75
Raisins, 1 tbsp	26	egg & tomato (1/2 of each)		65
Raspberries, 1 cup	70	fruit, mixed, 3 tbsp		150
Relish (see pickles)		gelatin (see gelatin)		
Rice		macaroni, 1/2 cup		167
brown, cooked, 1 cup	232	potato (see potato salad)		
white, cooked, 1 cup	223	tomato & cucumber		40
Rice mixes (commercial)		tuna		170
beef, 1 cup	320	Salami (see sausage)		
chicken, 1 cup	314	Salmon		
wild, 1 cup	282	Atlantic, 4 oz		230
Rice pudding, 1 cup	387	smoked, 4 oz		200
Rockfish, steamed, 4 oz	120	Salt		0
Rolls and buns		Sandwiches		
brown & serve	84	bacon, lettuce, tomato		280
Danish pastry, plain	317	bologna (2 oz)		248
hard roll, Kaiser	156	bologna & cheese		355
hoagie or submarine roll	392	cheese (2 oz)		314
frankfurter roll	119	cheese, cream/jelly		357
hamburger bun	119	chicken, 2 oz		196
sweet roll	180	Club		590
Root beer (see beverages)		corned beef, 2 oz		304
Rum (see beverages)		cucumber/tomato		124
Safflower oil (see oil)		egg, fried (1 egg)		206
Salad dressings (1 tbsp)		egg salad		280
blue cheese	76	ham, boiled, 2 oz		225
blue cheese, diet	12	ham, cheese		336
French	66	ham, deviled, 2 oz		291
French, diet	15	ham salad		320
Italian	83	hamburger, 2 oz		255
Italian, diet	8	hamburger/cheese		366
mayonnaise	101	lettuce/tomato		115
Roquefort	76	liverwurst		267
Roquefort, diet	12	peanut butter (2 tbsp)		292

peanut butter/cream cheese	348	Shortcake, strawberry	400
peanut butter/jelly	347	Shortening, 1 tbsp	100
roast beef, 2 oz	241	Shrimp	
salami, 2 oz	269	fresh, 4 oz	103
salmon, 2 oz	192	fried, 4 oz	256
tuna salad	280	Shrimp scampi, 6 in butter	265
turkey, 2 oz	200	Soft drinks (see beverages)	
Sardines, in oil, 4 oz	352	Sole, baked, 4 oz	90
Sauces (1 tbsp)		Soup (commercial, 1 cup)	
barbecue	17	asparagus, cream	65
butterscotch	100	bean	200
cheese, 1/4 cup	130	beef broth (bouillon)	31
chili	15	beef, consomme	70
chocolate	45	beef noodle	67
cream	35	celery, cream	86
fudge	50	chicken	75
Hollandaise, 1/4 cup	185	chicken, consomme	22
soy	10	chicken, cream	94
tartar	95	chicken, gumbo	55
tomato, canned, 1/4 cup	30	chicken, noodle	62
Worcestershire	10	chicken with rice	48
Sauerkraut, 1 cup	42	chicken vegetable	76
Sausage, cold cuts (1 oz)		clam chowder, Manhattan	76
bologna, 1 slice	40	clam chowder, New England	175
Braunschweiger	90	green pea	130
brown & serve sausage	120	minestrone	105
capicola	141	mushroom, cream	134
frankfurter, 1	170	onion	45
knockwurst	79	split pea	146
meatloaf	57	tomato	88
minced ham	65	turkey noodle	79
mortadella	89	vegetable	65
Polish sausage	86	vegetable beef	78
pork sausage	134	Soybeans, cooked, 1 cup	234
salami	128	Soybean curd (tofu), 1 oz	20
scrapple	61	Soybean oil (see oils)	
Scallions (see onions)		Soy sauce (see sauces)	
Scallops, 4 oz	127	Spaghetti	
Scrapple (see sausage)		dry, 4 oz	419
Sesame seeds, 1 tbsp	47	cooked, firm, 1 cup	192
Shad, baked, 4 oz	228	cooked, tender, 1 cup	155
Sherbet (see ice cream)		Spaghetti & meatballs, 1 cup	332
Shortbread (see cookies)		Spaghetti sauce/meat, 4 oz	109

Spanish rice, 1 cup	213	Tomato paste, canned, 4 oz	93
Spices	0	Toppings (see candy & sauces)	
Spinach, 1 cup	14	Tortilla, 5"	60
Squash		Trout, fresh, 4 oz	114
acorn, 1 squash	190	Tuna	
zucchini, sliced, 1 cup	22	canned, in oil, 4 oz	327
Stew (see beef & veg. stew)		canned, in water, 4 oz.	144
Strawberries, 1 cup	55	Tuna Salad (see salads)	
Stuffing, bread, 1/2 cup	350	Turkey, roasted, 4 oz	216
Sturgeon, cooked, 4 oz	180	Turnips, 1 cup	39
Succotash, 1 cup	158	Turnip greens, cooked, 1 cup	29
Sugar		Veal (4 oz)	
brown, packed, 1 cup	821	chuck	267
granulated, 1 cup	770	loin	265
granulated, 1 tbsp	46	rib roast	305
granulated, 1 lump (2 cubes)	19	Vegetables (see types)	
granulated, 1 packet	23	Vegetables, mixed, 1 cup	116
powdered, 1 cup	462	Venison, roasted	166
powdered, 1 tbsp	31	Vinegar, 1 cup	34
Sunflower seeds, hulled, 1 oz	159	Vodka (see beverages)	
Sweetpotatoes, baked, 4 oz	125	Waffles, 7" diam.	209
Swordfish, 4 oz	184	Walnuts, shelled, 1 oz	178
Syrups (see individual kinds)		Water chestnuts, 4 oz	69
		Watermelon	42
Tangerines	39	Wheat (see cereals, flours)	
Tapioca (see puddings)		Wheat germ, 1 tbsp	29
Tartar sauce (see sauces)		Whiskey (see beverages)	
Tea (see beverages)		Wine (see beverages)	
Tomatoes		Yeast, baker's, dry, 1 oz	80
fresh, 1 medium	27	Yogurt (1 cup)	
canned, 1 cup	51	plain, skimmed milk	123
puree, canned, 1 cup	100	plain, whole milk	153
Tomato juice, canned, 1 cup	46	coffee	200
Tomato juice, cocktail, 1 cup	51	strawberry	260
Tomato ketchup (see ketchup)		vanilla	200

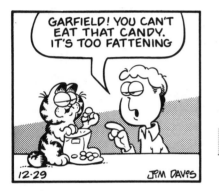
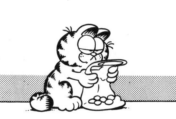
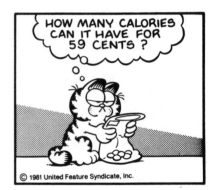

The LEARN™ Education Center

The LEARN Education Center was established to respond to the increasing demand for scientifically sound, state-of-the-art information, and professional training in weight control as well as other health and wellness areas. The Center is dedicated to the continuing development of support materials in the area of weight control such as audio and video tapes, newsletters, and expert counseling support.

The Center has available *The LEARN Program for Weight Control*, by Kelly D. Brownell, Ph.D. This manual has been written in consultation with colleagues in nutrition, exercise physiology, psychology and relapse prevention. The 1990 edition of the manual includes 208 pages of detailed information in the five areas shown below, hence the **LEARN** title.

L   Lifestyle (Behavior Modification)

E   Exercise (Body Fitness)

A   Attitudes (Cognitive Factors, Relapse Prevention)

R   Relationships (Social Support, Family Factors)

N   Nutrition

This manual is a step-by-step guide for persons losing weight. It contains an Orientation, 16 lessons, self-assessment questions, several appendices and a calorie guide. Each lesson has a thorough discussion of the material, charts and illustrations including forms for recording food intake, exercise and behavior change. The manual is written to be upbeat, encouraging and instructive. It can be used in conjunction with professional assistance or stand alone as a weight loss guide and has been used in individual patient counseling, medical settings, work site programs, weight loss clinics, rehabilitation programs and other settings.

Serving as a training guide for professionals, the manual is used by dietitians, physicians, nurses, health educators, exercise instructors, psychologists, counselors and other professionals.

The new edition of The LEARN Manual (copyright 1990), in now in print and available. Not available in book stores, the manual may be obtained by calling our toll-free number listed in the next section.

ORDERING INFORMATION

This manual and the **Personal Maintenance Kit** are not available in bookstores and may be obtained only through The LEARN Education Center at the address listed below. You may write or call the toll free number to obtain current pricing and shipping charges for this manual as well as other materials and publications. Discounts are available for bulk orders.

For your ordering convenience, a toll-free number may be called 24 hours a day. In addition, the Center accepts MasterCard and VISA telephone orders for all publications and training courses. These services have been established to help us respond quickly to your needs. All orders are shipped within 24 hours, and next-day and 2nd-day UPS deliveries are available.

As you use our publications, we sincerely welcome any comments for improvement. We encourage you to tell us how we are doing.

We are continually developing new materials and publications, such as newsletters, audio and video tapes, and training courses in weight loss as well as other health and wellness areas. Call or write to be added to our mailing list.

For ordering and general information, please write or call us at:

The LEARN Education Center
1555 W. Mockingbird Lane, Suite 203
Dallas, Texas 75235

Our toll-free number is **1-800-736-READ**
In Dallas **214-637-7700**
Our fax number is **214-637-0529**

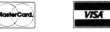

About The Authors

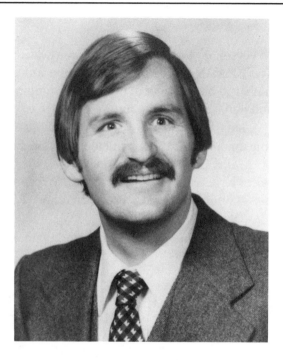

Kelly D. Brownell, Ph.D. is an internationally known expert on weight control. He received training at Purdue University, Rutgers University, and Brown University, and is currently Professor, Department of Psychiatry, University of Pennsylvania School of Medicine, and Co-Director of the Obesity Research Clinic. He has written ten books and over 100 research paper in scientific journals, and holds appointments on 10 editorial boards. Dr. Brownell has received awards from the American Psychological Association and the New York Academy of Sciences, and has been awarded research grants from the National Institute of Health, the MacArthur Foundation, and the National Institute of Mental Health. He has been the President of the Society of Behavioral Medicine, the Division of Health Psychology of the American Psychological Association and the Association for the Advancement of Behavior Therapy. He has been an advisor to the U.S. Navy, American Airlines, Johnson & Johnson and other organizations. He has appeared on *Good Morning America*, the *Today Show*, *Nova* and *20/20*, and his work has been featured in the *New York Times*, *Washington Post*, *Glamour*, *Redbook*, *Family Circle*, *Vogue*, and other publications.

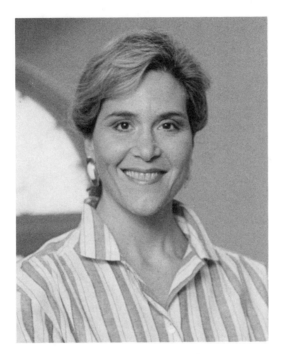

Judith Rodin, Ph.D. is known world-wide for her work on obesity, eating disorders and aging. She received training at the University of Pennsylvania, Columbia University and the University of California-Irvine, and is currently the Philip R. Allen Professor and Chair of the Psychology Department at Yale University and Professor of Medicine and Psychiatry at Yale School of Medicine. She has written six books and over 150 research articles and chapters in scientific journals. She is Chief Editor of the journal *Appetite* and holds appointments on seven editorial boards. Dr. Rodin has received awards from the American Psychological Association and the Gerontological Society of America, and has been awarded research grants from the National Institute of Health, the National Science Foundation, the MacArthur Foundation, and the Schimper Foundation. She is President of the Society of Behavioral Medicine and has been President of the Eastern Psychological Association and the Division of Health Psychology of the American Psychological Association. She currently chairs the MacArthur Foundation Research Network on the Determinants and Consequences of Health Promoting and Health Damaging Behavior. She has co-hosted the PBS television series *Bodywatch* and has appeared on *Good Morning America*, the *Today Show*, *Nova* and *Donahue*. Her work has been featured in the *New York Times*, *Washington Post*, *Glamour*, *Vogue*, *Reader's Digest*, *American Health*, *Psychology Today* and other publications.